Prentice Hall Health

review manual

for the First Responder

Joseph J. Mistovich, M.Ed., NREMT-P
Chairperson and Professor
Department of Health Professions
Youngstown State University
Youngstown, Ohio

PEARSON

Prentice Hall

Upper Saddle River, New Jersey 07458

Library of Congress Cataloging-in-Publication Data

Mistovich, Joseph J.
  Prentice Hall Health review manual for the first responder/Joseph J. Mistovich.
  p. cm.—(Prentice Hall Health review series)
  Includes index.
  ISBN 0-13-118439-3
    1. Medical emergencies—Examinations, questions, etc. 2. Emergency medical
technicians—Examinations, questions, etc. 3. First aid in illness and injury—
Examinations, questions, etc. [DNLM: 1. Emergency Medical Services—
methods—Examination Questions.
    2. Emergency Medical Technicians—Examination Questions.
WX 18.2 M678p 2005] I. Title: Review manual for the first responder. II.
Title. III. Series.

RC86.7.M56 2005
616.02′5′076—dc22   2004011039

Publisher: Julie Levin Alexander
Publisher's Assistant: Regina Bruno
Executive Editor: Marlene McHugh Pratt
Senior Managing Editor for Development: Lois Berlowitz
Project Manager: Andrea Edwards
Assistant Editor: Monica Moosang
Senior Marketing Manager: Katrin Beacom
Channel Marketing Manager: Rachele Strober
Marketing Coordinator: Michael Sirinides
Director of Production and Manufacturing: Bruce Johnson
Managing Editor for Production: Patrick Walsh
Production Liaison: Faye Gemmellaro
Production Editor: Robert Saley/nSight, Inc.
Manufacturing Manager: Ilene Sanford
Manufacturing Buyer: Pat Brown
Creative Director: Cheryl Asherman
Senior Design Coordinator: Christopher Weigand
Cover/Interior Designer: Janice Bielawa
Composition: Laserwords
Printing and Binding: Courier Westford
Cover Printer: Coral Graphics

Studentaid.ed.gov, the U.S. Department of Education's website on college planning assistance, is a valuable tool for anyone intending to pursue higher education. Designed to help students at all stages of schooling, including international students, returning students, and parents, it is a guide to the financial aid process. The website presents information on applying to and attending college as well as on funding your education and repaying loans. It also provides links to useful resources, such as state education agency contact information, assistance in filling out financial aid forms, and an introduction to various forms of student aid.

10 9 8 7 6 5 4 3 2
ISBN 0-13-118439-3

This book is dedicated to the memory of my father, who provided me with the love and encouragement that allowed me to pursue my dreams. He will always be my inspiration to continue living life to its fullest, no matter what obstacles I encounter. To my beautiful wife Andrea, who continues to be my greatest supporter and best friend. To my wonderful children, Katie, Kristyn, Chelsea, Morgan, and Kara, for helping me get through another project. Your energy, hugs, kisses, and smiles make every day so much brighter! I love you all dearly!

Joseph J. Mistovich

Contents

Preface

The purpose of this review manual is to help prepare you for examinations in your First Responder course and your certification examination. The manual consists of a series of self-assessment sections that can identify your strengths and weaknesses in relation to the information you are studying. If you are a currently certified First Responder, this manual can serve as a refresher tool itself or as a method to determine where your knowledge has deteriorated and your need for specific review.

The **Review Manual for the First Responder** consists of multiple-choice type items that are organized according to the U.S. Department of Transportation's (D.O.T.'s) National Standard First Responder Curriculum. Enhancement questions are included that are supplemental to the D.O.T. curriculum. Every item has a corresponding answer and rationale. In addition, every item, with the exception of those that are considered "enhancement items," is referenced to a specific D.O.T. objective. This reference can be found after the module questions in the "answers & rationales" section. Answers and rationales marked with an asterisk are supplemental to the D.O.T. curriculum.

You will also find that many of the answers and rationales are followed by page references that correspond to Brady's First Responder textbooks, which will allow you to find more specific information on a topic or concept. "FR7" refers to *First Responder*, 7e (Bergeron, Bizjak, Krause, Le Baudour). "FRASA" refers to *First Responder: A Skills Approach*, 7e (Limmer, Karren, Hafen).

The author and manuscript reviewers all have extensive knowledge and experience as EMS educators. The items were developed in a "teacher-made test format" to allow you to test your knowledge and understanding of the material. When compiled into a series of sections, the items serve as a self-assessment tool to identify particular strengths and weaknesses in your knowledge and understanding of the information. This allows you to concentrate on specific sections that have been identified as a weakness. A comprehensive examination has also been provided to allow you to test your knowledge at the First Responder level.

This manual should be used as a tool to better prepare you for your examinations. However, there is no better preparation than studying and understanding the information that has been presented to you in your course. To best ensure your success on the examination, I encourage you to study first until you feel confident that you know the information and then use this manual as a self-assessment to determine how well you know the information. When you have identified areas of weakness, do not simply study the manual or review items. Go back and study the information presented to you, study the textbook, and use other sources to better understand the information. Once you again feel confident you know the material, retest yourself using the review manual to determine if you are better prepared for that section.

I hope this manual assists you in preparing for your examination. However, when it comes time to manage a patient in the prehospital environment, there is no time for preparation. You must draw on your existing knowledge and skills to successfully and efficiently treat the patient. Thus, it is imperative to good patient care that you are truly prepared not only to pass that examination but to take care of each and every patient you encounter to the best of your ability. Good luck in your EMS endeavors!

Joseph J. Mistovich

Reviewers

We would like to thank the following reviewers for their helpful comments and insights in the preparation of this review manual.

John B. Booth
Captain, R.F.C.
Fire-Rescue
Harbor Springs, MI

William Clark
Mississippi EMT Association
Escalawpa VFD
Moss Point, MS

Scott Garrett
Director of Education
Upstate EMS Council
Greenville, SC

Douglas R. Smith, MA, EMT-P, I/C
Platinum Educational Group
Jenison, MI

Introduction

SUCCESS ACROSS THE BOARDS: THE PRENTICE HALL HEALTH REVIEW SERIES

Prentice Hall Health is pleased to present the ***Review Manual for the First Responder*** as part of a review series on the various EMS education levels. The authoritative text gives you expert help in preparing for certification examinations.

ABOUT THE BOOK:

- **Review Manual for the First Responder:** This manual has been designed to help students prepare for the written course and certification examinations. It can also be used as a review for currently certified First Responders. A total of 1,000 multiple-choice items are organized by the sections covered in the D.O.T.'s National Standard First Responder Curriculum. The multiple-choice items are similar to those found on teacher-made and certifying exams. Working through these items will help you assess your strengths and weaknesses in each section.

- **D.O.T. Objectives:** A D.O.T. objective reference number, located after the module questions in the "answers & rationales" section, allows you to refer back to the specific D.O.T. Curriculum objective that the item was written from. This will allow you to seek more information for each item from popular textbooks written to the D.O.T objectives. The enhancement material tests knowledge that is beyond the D.O.T. objectives; therefore, those respective answers and rationales do not have objective reference numbers. These are marked with an asterisk.

- **Answers and Rationales:** Correct answers and comprehensive rationales are provided and assist you in better understanding each item. Rationales for incorrect answers are typically presented so that you may also learn why that answer is incorrect.

- **Page References:** Page references to Brady's First Responder textbooks, *First Responder*, 7e, and *First Responder: A Skills Approach*, 6e, are included after many rationales to allow you to find further information on a subject.

- **First Responder Self-Assessment Practice Test:** A comprehensive self-assessment test is provided as a practice exam to test your overall knowledge of the information.

So, you're getting ready for an exam. Congratulations for making it to this point! Now let's help you make the next step—doing your best on this exam. Some people find test taking unsettling, while many consider tests unnerving and even scary! Use this book as an opportunity for personal preparation and information review and to practice the techniques covered in the exam.

PHYSICAL PREPARATION

The key to maximizing your potential on a test is to be at your personal best. Along with mental preparation, physical preparation should be included in a good study strategy. Physical preparation includes getting adequate rest and exercising. It also includes eating a balanced meal the night before and the morning of the exam. Your brain works best when it has access to a supply of glucose. So fruits, grains, vegetables, and pasta are important foods. Try to avoid caffeine and foods with high sugar content on the morning of the exam. These foods provide a short burst of energy, but when they are used up, the slump will significantly reduce your ability to function.

Try some physical exercise the days before the exam but not to the point of exhaustion. Increasing cardiovascular perfusion will also increase perfusion to the brain. More oxygen circulating in the brain can only be good, right? Exercise is also an outlet for stress, making it easier to get a good night's sleep.

INFORMATION REVIEW

Against popular belief, preparing for the exam should not include extensive studying. You've been studying for months, you know the material, and cramming now will probably cause an intellectual shutdown. Review the material for short periods of time, and take frequent breaks. Try study groups of

three to five people for review; the active discussion will be an excellent way to reinforce the material and retain the information.

Although knowing the material is essential, physical preparation is equally important. Remember, review only in brief intervals, use a study group, and don't cram.

TAKING THE EXAMINATION

An exam is not written by happenstance; it's an art and a science. Each time you take an exam, it's a chance to evaluate your knowledge, as well as to hone your test-taking skills. A test might seem hard, but exams are generally built to measure **minimum** competency. Certification or recertification exams are usually not designed to test total knowledge, ability to expertly function in the field, or even your level of professionalism. They are an attempt to evaluate your reading comprehension and judgment.

There are two basic kinds of questions found on most certification exams: multiple choice and true/false. Each of these questions is built in a specific way to test your ability and your knowledge. Knowing how the questions are constructed may help you during the exam.

Multiple-choice exams consist of two parts: stems and answers. A stem is the actual question part, and the list of answers that follows are called distracters. Distracters are designed to (what else?) distract you from the correct response. Multiple-choice questions require your knowledge, judgment, and expertise to answer the question. Hint: use the process of elimination.

When answering a multiple-choice question, read the question and all of the answers first. Then begin the process of elimination, starting with the most incorrect and sorting your way through until you're left with one or two possible answers. Got a problem picking from those? Then reread the stem. If it would make it easier, then rephrase the question, looking for key words that give you a hint about the answer. Don't forget to look at the grammar; is the stem in plural form or singular? Whatever process you use, try not to spend more than 2 minutes on any one question.

You may find a topic is covered in several consecutive questions. In this case, be sure all your answers are similar and seem to fit together. It might be helpful to use the previous answers to validate each new set of choices. Another option is to check the next question because sometimes the answer, or a strong hint to one question, is the stem of the following questions. Remember, when reading multiple-choice responses, the correct answer may be the most comprehensive choice—you know, the one that combines several of the other answers or includes more details.

If the exam contains true/false questions, remember that statements containing absolute terms such as "never," "always," and "only" will usually be false. Very little of medicine, or life itself, is absolute. Statements that contain words such as "maybe" or "sometimes" tend to be true. These are some hints that may help you when reading true/false questions.

The scientific part of test building is putting all the information into questions. The key is to read each question carefully. Try not to scan because you miss important key words such as **incorrect** or **not**, which cause you to waste time or, more important, miss the answer. Be prudent, pace yourself, and use patience—your all-important "three Ps."

WRAPPING UP

You know how people say to go with your first hunch? Well, they're right. Your brain makes immediate connections based on stored information and your experience. Don't be afraid that the answer is wrong just because you didn't go through all the usual steps of logic. Research shows that first impressions tend to be correct.

It's okay to choose the same letter answer two or three times in a row. The answers are put into a question at random, so it could be that the same letter shows up as being correct up to five times. Don't change your answer if you have chosen the same letter more than once.

Well, you have done the most you can by participating in class, practicing your skills, and reading your material. You know it all by now, so trying to teach yourself the curriculum just won't work and ultimately your patients will suffer. Trust yourself and your abilities. Practice some of the tips in this section as you proceed through this book. In the days before the exam, remember to eat well, exercise, and get sleep. Good luck.

1 Preparatory

module objectives

Questions in this module relate to D.O.T.
objectives 1-1.1 to 1-5.5.

1. Which of the following is **not** one of the classic components of an emergency medical services (EMS) system identified by the "Technical Assistance Program Assessment Standards" provided by the National Highway Traffic Safety Administration?
   A. regulation and policy
   B. equipment acquisition
   C. communications
   D. resource management

2. Safety at the scene is the primary responsibility of the:
   A. incident commander.
   B. individual First Responder.
   C. ranking fire officer.
   D. scene safety officer.

3. You arrive on the scene of a shooting in a housing project and find a patient lying on the sidewalk in a pool of blood. A large, gaping open wound to the upper thigh is spurting blood. The patient is still clutching a pistol while thrashing around and screaming. Your first action should be to:
   A. immediately apply direct pressure to the open thigh wound.
   B. restrain the patient and attempt to control the weapon.
   C. retreat and clear the bystanders from around the patient.
   D. attempt to knock the gun from the patient's hand.

4. Medical oversight of First Responders in an EMS system is:
   A. provided by a supervising nurse in the emergency department.
   B. provided by the agency's training or education staff.
   C. the ultimate responsibility of a physician system medical director.
   D. provided by the use of well-defined treatment protocols.

5. The First Responder is **not** responsible for which of the following at the scene of a medical emergency?
   A. assessing for immediate life threats to the patient
   B. writing and submitting reports regarding the incident
   C. determining a diagnosis of the patient
   D. conducting a physical examination of the patient

SCENARIO

Questions 6–9 refer to the following scenario:

You are dispatched to a residence for a patient who dialed 911, spoke inappropriate words, and quickly hung up prior to providing any coherent information. You respond and arrive on the scene to find a patient who is confused and exhibiting the signs and symptoms of a low blood sugar level. You determine in your assessment that the patient is alert but confused and is able to swallow adequately. You place the patient on oxygen and contact medical oversight by radio to get permission to administer a tube of oral glucose.

6. What type of call delivery system did the patient initially access to contact EMS?
   A. a non-911 call system with caller ID
   B. a basic 911 call delivery system
   C. an enhanced 911 call delivery system
   D. a computer-aided dispatch system

7. Your treatment of placing the patient on oxygen is an example of a(n):
   A. direct medical control.
   B. off-line medical control order.
   C. immediate medical control order.
   D. concurrent medical control order.

8. A written document that provides you with the ability to function using both off-line and on-line medical oversight orders is referred to as:
   A. protocol.
   B. quality improvement.
   C. base station orders.
   D. quality assurance orders.

9. Which of the following would be considered an example of an on-line medical director order?
   A. initial assessment of the patient
   B. application of oxygen via a nonrebreather mask
   C. assessment of the blood pressure
   D. administration of oral glucose by mouth

10. When dealing with a patient diagnosed as having terminal lung cancer, you notice that the patient is silent, distant, and sad. The emotional stage the patient most likely is exhibiting is:
    A. denial.
    B. bargaining.
    C. acceptance.
    D. depression.

11. A terminally ill patient who is coping with his disease and is prepared to die is likely to be exhibiting:
    A. denial.
    B. bargaining.
    C. acceptance.
    D. depression.

12. If your family and friends lack an understanding of EMS and your responsibilities as a First Responder, it will most likely:
    A. lead to a stressful relationship.
    B. relieve them of undue worry while you are working.
    C. lessen their frustrations with the requirements of your job.
    D. reduce their fear of separation.

13. A version of Critical Incident Stress Debriefing (CISD) that is held within 1 to 4 hours following a critical incident is called a(n):
    A. review.
    B. defusing.
    C. follow-up.
    D. incident recap.

14. You are treating a trauma patient with a large laceration to his upper extremity that is spurting blood. You should use all of the following body substance isolation equipment **except:**
    A. eyewear with side shields.
    B. latex or vinyl gloves.
    C. protective clothing or gown.
    D. a high efficiency particulate air (HEPA) respirator.

15. Your legal right to function as a First Responder may be contingent upon:
    A. acquiring medical direction.
    B. maintaining malpractice insurance.
    C. mastery of the necessary skills.
    D. acting in an ethical manner.

16. Permission must be obtained prior to rendering care to a patient. This is termed:
    A. consent.
    B. an "acknowledgment of care."
    C. EMS treatment recognition.
    D. a pre-care protocol.

17. You arrive on the scene and find a 45-year-old patient lying on the street corner who responds to your questions with inappropriate words and phrases. You should immediately:
    A. assess your patient and initiate emergency care.
    B. attempt to determine the patient's name, address, and phone number.
    C. contact the police and wait for their consent to initiate care.
    D. cease assessment or treatment until expressed consent is obtained.

18. Which patient is most likely capable of refusing treatment?

    A. a patient who flexes his arms across his chest when you apply a painful stimuli

    B. a patient who appears to be intoxicated

    C. a patient who gestures you away when obtaining consent

    D. a patient who speaks with inappropriate words

19. You are assessing a 62-year-old female patient who complains of chest pain. Initially, she agreed to allow you to treat her; however, she now refuses treatment. Her husband requests that you continue to treat her. You initiated treatment prior to her refusing treatment. Given these circumstances you should:

    A. continue treatment and contact EMS for quick transport.

    B. cease additional treatment and gain written permission from her husband.

    C. immediately reevaluate her level of competency.

    D. restrain her, continue to treat, and then contact medical control for additional assistance.

20. A patient refuses treatment. She is alert and oriented and answers questions appropriately. She refuses to sign a "Release from Liability Form." Your best action would be to:

    A. have both you and your partner sign for the patient.

    B. leave the scene and have your partner sign as a witness to the refusal.

    C. leave the scene quickly and advise the husband to call back if needed.

    D. have the husband sign the form as a witness to the wife's refusal.

21. A patient continues to refuse treatment after assessment and explanation of the consequences of refusing care. Prior to departing the scene you should:

    A. say nothing and avoid any eye contact with the family and patient.

    B. try again to persuade the patient to accept treatment.

    C. prepare to transport the patient in spite of her repeated refusals.

    D. describe complications of refusal to the patient, using the appropriate medical terminology.

22. You are asked to accompany the EMS team during transport of a patient. When you arrive at the hospital, the emergency department is extremely busy. The ward clerk yells out to move the patient to any of the rooms that are empty. While you and the EMS team move the patient to a hospital bed, you are toned out for another emergency. On your way out of the emergency department, you can only find the ward clerk to tell her that the patient is in room 2A. You then respond to your next call. This action could result in:

    A. a continuous quality improvement investigation for improper consent.

    B. a charge of abandonment by the patient you just transported.

    C. a charge of negligence by the patient that you are responding to.

    D. better continuation of care delivered by the emergency department.

23. A woman contacts you who states she is the grandmother of a minor patient you treated at the school playground today. She requests information related to the assessment findings and care of the patient. She states she is the patient's legal guardian. The best action for you to take is to:

    A. provide the information requested and document the conversation.

    B. provide the information; there is no need to document the conversation.

C. provide the information and then contact your supervisor.

D. not release the information until a release form is obtained.

24. Your patient has a deformity to the midshaft of the forearm. He most likely has suffered an injury to which of the following bones?
    A. femur
    B. patella
    C. fibula
    D. radius

25. Which of the following would be an action performed by a skeletal muscle?
    A. contraction of the left ventricle
    B. constriction of a blood vessel
    C. movement of the fingers
    D. movement of food down the small intestine

26. If the muscles of the upper airway relax in an unresponsive patient, the tongue will cause an obstruction at the level of the:
    A. pharynx.
    B. nasopharynx.
    C. trachea.
    D. carina.

27. During inhalation:
    A. the diaphragm moves downward and the chest moves outward.
    B. the diaphragm moves downward and the chest moves inward.
    C. the diaphragm moves upward and the chest moves outward.
    D. the diaphragm moves upward and the chest moves inward.

28. Which of the following would most likely occur if the epiglottis were to malfunction?
    A. air would be directed into the larynx and trachea
    B. blood would be diverted away from the heart and lungs

C. secretions may enter the trachea and get into the lungs

D. the left ventricle would not eject an adequate amount of blood

29. The most common cause of cardiac arrest in infants and young children is due to:
    A. cardiac rhythm problems.
    B. liver and kidney failure.
    C. congential heart defects undetected at birth.
    D. an airway obstruction or respiratory problem.

30. Which of the following would be the best direct indicator of the function of the left ventricle?
    A. diastolic blood pressure
    B. pulse quality
    C. respiratory rate
    D. orientation of the patient

31. After blood is circulated and oxygenated in the lungs, it is returned next to which chamber of the heart?
    A. right atrium
    B. left atrium
    C. right ventricle
    D. left ventricle

32. Which of the following pulses should be assessed in an infant?
    A. carotid
    B. brachial
    C. radial
    D. femoral

33. Oxygen and carbon dioxide are exchanged with the cells throughout the body in the:
    A. arteries.
    B. veins.
    C. ventricles.
    D. capillaries.

34. Which of the following is a component of the central nervous system?
    A. sensory nerves
    B. peripheral nerves
    C. brain
    D. motor nerves

35. In response to cold, the skin helps maintain body core temperature by:
    A. constricting vessels.
    B. producing sweat.
    C. dilating vessels.
    D. secreting oil from glands.

36. While lifting a patient from the ground, your back should be:
    A. curved slightly outward and not locked.
    B. curved slightly inward in a locked position.
    C. in a relaxed position of comfort.
    D. parallel to the ground and in a locked position.

37. Which technique best protects your back from injury when carrying a heavy object?
    A. lifting with a twisting motion
    B. hyperextending your back by leaning backwards
    C. keeping the weight as close to your body as possible
    D. keeping your back in a relaxed unlocked position

38. Your patient, who is alert and oriented and has no critical illness or injury, is on the second floor of his house in the back bedroom. The best possible method to move the patient down the steps to the ground floor is by:
    A. securing the patient in a seated position in a stair chair.
    B. using the stretcher with the carriage in the up position.
    C. securing the patient to a long backboard with immobilization straps.
    D. carrying the patient using a two-person extremity lift.

39. To help prevent injury when performing a one-handed carrying technique, which of the following should you avoid?
    A. keeping your abdominal muscles tight
    B. bending at the hips
    C. positioning your back in a locked position
    D. leaning too far to the opposite side

40. The preferred method to move a responsive, non-injured patient down steps is by the use of a(n):
    A. long spine board.
    B. ambulance stretcher.
    C. stair chair.
    D. vest-type immobilization device.

41. Which of the following is correct and should be used to aid against injury when performing a logroll?
    A. Use your shoulder muscles whenever possible.
    B. Lean toward the patient from your waist, not your hips.
    C. Use your lower back muscles to support your weight.
    D. Keep your back in a relaxed position by leaning back.

42. Whenever possible, when moving an object it should be:
    A. pushed rather than pulled.
    B. lifted from the waist.
    C. pulled as low as possible to the ground.
    D. lifted as far from the body as possible.

43. In which of the following situations would an emergency move be appropriate to move a patient?
    A. to shield him or her from curious onlookers (protect modesty)
    B. to gain access to another patient that is critically injured

C. to allow law enforcement officers to direct traffic through the scene

D. to provide adequate space for the traffic investigation team

44. You arrive on the scene and find a 34-year-old male patient lying in a hospital bed in his home. The dispatcher notifies you that the patient is HIV positive and has AIDS. When you arrive at the scene, you are greeted at the door by his sister. She informs you that the patient is coughing up blood-tinged sputum, has been sweating at night profusely, and has lost weight recently. Your next immediate action should be to:

A. refuse to enter the scene because of your risk of contracting HIV.

B. put on gloves, eye protection, and a HEPA respirator before entering.

C. apply a surgical mask to the patient to reduce the risk of droplet spread.

D. contact medical direction to determine if you should enter the scene.

45. You arrive on the scene and find a 20-year-old male patient who has been involved in an auto crash. Upon assessment, you note the patient cannot tell you what date it is, where he is, or whom he is with. The patient refuses to let you examine him further and refuses any emergency care. You should:

A. have the patient sign a refusal form and then leave the scene.

B. turn the patient over to the police on the scene and then leave.

C. begin to administer emergency care to the patient using restraints if necessary.

D. instruct the police to contact a family member of the patient to gain consent for treatment.

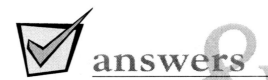

answers & rationales

Following each rationale, you will find a reference to the corresponding D.O.T. objective. A rationale marked with an asterisk denotes material supplemental to the First Responder curriculum. Also included after each rationale are references to where the question topic may be covered in Brady First Responder textbooks. **"FR7" refers to *First Responder*, 7e** (Bergeron, Bizjak, Krause, Le Baudour). **"FRASA" refers to *First Responder: A Skills Approach*, 7e** (Limmer, Karren, Hafen).

1.

B. Equipment acquisition is not one of the recommended standards identified by the "Technical Assistance Program Assessment Standards" or classic components of an EMS System. The ten standards are regulation and policy, resource management, human resources and training, transportation, facilities, communications, public information and education, medical direction, trauma systems, and evaluation. (1-1.1) (FR7 p. 2; FRASA p. 7)

2.

B. Each individual who responds to the scene is responsible for his or her own personal safety. Other rescuers have specific responsibilities for assuring a safe rescue operation by observing for unsafe activities. This does not relieve the First Responder from the responsibility of assuring personal safety at all times. (1-1.2) (FR7 p. 8; FRASA p. 8)

3.

C. Personal safety is your primary role and responsibility, while safety of the others members of the crew, patient, and bystanders is your second priority. Once safety is assured, the patient's needs become your first priority. (1-1.2) (FR7 p. 8; FRASA pp. 23–24)

4.

C. The physician medical director of an EMS system is responsible for all patient care and clinical aspects of system management. This includes all levels of care provided from First Responder to EMT-Paramedic. The other individuals listed in the question do play roles in medical direction, but they do not assume ultimate responsibility. (1-1.3) (FR7 p. 5; FRASA p. 9)

5.

C. The First Responder is not responsible for determining the diagnosis of the patient. The First Responder's responsibilities are to gain access to the patient, perform an assessment and provide emergency care, assist with continued care of the patient once other EMS personnel arrive on the scene, and write and maintain records as necessary. (1-1.2) (FR7 p. 6; FRASA pp. 8–9)

6.

C. An enhanced 911 system allows for both automated number identification (ANI) and automated location identification (ALI). This provides the public service answering point call taker with the phone number, name, and address of the residence at which the call was placed. Once the contact is made, regardless of whether the patient hangs up the phone or not, the information is displayed at the call taker's terminal. A fire, police, or medical response can be made based on that information even without the patient uttering a word. (1-1.1) (FR7 p. 3; FRASA p. 4)

7.

B. There are two types of medical oversight. Direct medical control, also known as on-line, base station, immediate, or concurrent, is provided by directly communicating with medical control via radio, phone, or actual contact at the time of the call. Indirect medical control, also known as off-line, retrospective, or prospective, is provided by written protocols. There is no communication at the time of the call when using off-line or indirect medical oversight. (1-1.4) (FR7 p. 5; FRASA p. 9)

8.

A. Your protocol is a set of written medical directives provided by the medical director that outlines what treatment can be provided as on-line or with direct communication with the medical control physician and what treatment can be provided as off-line or without direct communication with the medical control physician. (1-1.4) (FR7 p. 5; FRASA p. 9)

9.

D. Since the First Responder was required to contact medical control to get permission to administer the oral glucose, it is considered an on-line medical control order. The First Responder was not required to contact medical control for permission to apply and administer oxygen, thus it is considered an off-line order. Assessment of the patient did not require direct on-line permission from medical control. (1-1.4) (FR7 pp. 5–6; FRASA p. 9)

10.

D. The patient may display five various emotional stages associated with death and dying. Depression is associated with silent, distant, sad, and despairing behavior. (1-2.2) (FR7 p. 39; FRASA p. 26)

11.

C. Acceptance is when the patient appears to accept death. He or she typically is no longer afraid to die. (1-2.2) (FR7 p. 39; FRASA p. 26)

12.

A. A lack of understanding of your role and responsibility as First Responder will likely lead to a stressful relationship with family and friends. Other stress responses by family and friends may include fear of separation or of being ignored, worry about on-call situations, frustration with the inability to plan, and frustration with your desire to share your experiences. (1-2.4) (FR7 p. 36; FRASA p. 28)

13.

B. A formal CISD is held within 24 to 72 hours after a critical incident. A team of peer counselors guides rescuers through varied phases of discussion. Defusing is a version of CISD that is held within 1 to 4 hours following a critical incident. The defusion is attended by those directly involved in the incident. (1-2.6) (FR7 p. 41; FRASA p. 29)

14.

D. A HEPA respirator or N-95 mask is used to filter out the organism responsible for transmitting tuberculosis. Unless your patient is exhibiting signs and symptoms of tuberculosis, there is no need to wear a HEPA respirator. Vinyl or latex gloves, eye wear with side shields, and gowns are appropriate to wear when contact with spurting blood or splashes is suspected. (1-2.9) (FR7 p. 44; FRASA pp. 20–21)

15.

A. Your legal right to function as a First Responder is contingent upon acquiring medical direction through protocols and standing orders. Without medical direction, you cannot function. It is an ethical responsibility to strive to achieve mastery of your skills. (1-3.1) (FR7 p. 19; FRASA p. 35)

16.

A. Consent is the permission to care for a patient. Consent must be obtained from all patients prior to treatment. There are three primary forms of consent: expressed, implied, and consent to treat a minor or mentally incompetent adult. (1-3.3) (FR7 p. 21–23; FRASA p. 36)

17.

A. Based on the concept of implied consent, you should immediately assess your patient and initiate emergency care. (1-3.4) (FR7 p. 23; FRASA p. 36)

18.

C. A competent adult has the right to refuse treatment. A patient with an altered mental status or under the influence of alcohol or drugs may be considered incompetent. Incompetence would depend upon the extent to which the drugs or alcohol are clouding the patient's judgment. Oral refusal or actions (such as gestures) that imply refusal are considered valid forms of patient refusal. (1-3.6) (FR7 p. 21; FRASA p. 36)

19.

C. When dealing with refusal issues, it is important to determine the patient's competency or lack of competency. A competent adult has the right to refuse treatment or to withdraw from treatment once it has started. If you are unsure as to whether or not the patient is competent, contact medical direction. (1-3.6) (FR7 p. 21; FRASA p. 37)

answers & rationales

20.

D. The best answer is to have the patient's husband sign as a witness to the refusal. The witnessed refusal form becomes a part of the legal documentation of the patient's refusal. You must document all aspects of the patient encounter to include history obtained and physical exam findings. Also, document your attempts at treatment and transport. (1-3.6) (FR7 p. 22; FRASA pp. 38–39)

21.

B. Before leaving any patient who has refused treatment or transport, always try one last time to persuade the patient to accept emergency care and transport. (1-3.6) (FR7 p. 21; FRASA p. 38)

22.

B. Termination of care without assuring the proper continuation of care by a competent practitioner can result in a charge of abandonment. If in the hospital, proper transfer of care to an equally or more highly qualified health care practitioner must occur. Failure to properly transfer that care can result in a charge of abandonment. (1-3.7) (FR7 p. 27; FRASA p. 39)

23.

D. Releasing confidential information requires a written release form signed by the patient or a legal guardian. Do not release confidential information about the patient to someone claiming to be a legal guardian. Guardianship must be established. (1-3.9) (FR7 p. 28; FRASA p. 41)

24.

D. There are two bones that comprise the forearm: the radius and the ulna. The radius is on the thumb side and the ulna is on the little finger side. (1-4.3) (FR7 p. 357; FRASA pp. 55–56)

25.

C. Skeletal muscle is responsible for voluntary movement. Smooth muscle is found in organs, blood vessels, respiratory tract, and other tubular structures in the body. Cardiac muscle is found in the heart. Smooth and cardiac muscle are under involuntary control. (1-4.3) (FR7 p. 61; FRASA p. 56)

26.

A. When the muscles of the upper airway relax, the tongue will fall back and create an airway occlusion at the level of the pharynx. The nasopharynx begins at the nares and ends at the level of the pharynx. The tongue cannot occlude the nasopharynx. (1-4.1) (FRASA p. 56)

27.

A. During inhalation, the diaphragm and intercostal muscles contract. This contraction of muscles moves the diaphragm downward, and the chest wall is lifted outward. The increase in the chest cavity size causes the pressure inside the chest cavity to become negative, causing air to flow into the lungs. (1-4.1) (FR7 pp. 98–99; FRASA p. 56)

28.

C. The epiglottis is a flap of cartilaginous tissue that is responsible for covering the opening to the larynx when a patient swallows. If the epiglottis were to malfunction, secretions, blood, food, or liquids may enter the larynx and trachea and may eventually enter the lungs. If food, liquid, blood, vomitus, or secretions are allowed to enter the lungs, the patient may exhibit signs and symptoms of respiratory distress. (1-4.1) (FR7 p. 100; FRASA p. 56)

29.

D. The most common cause of cardiac arrest in infants and young children is an airway obstruction or respiratory failure. (1-4.1) (FR7 p. 108; FRASA p. 58)

30.

B. The pulse is generated by a wave of blood being ejected by the left ventricle. Pulse quality, or the strength of the pulse, would be the best direct indicator of the left ventricle function. Thus, a strong pulse would indicate good pumping function of the left ventricle. (1-4.2) (FR7 p. 541; FRASA p. 58)

31.

B. After being oxygenated in the lungs, the blood travels through the pulmonary vein and enters the left atrium. From the left atrium, the blood is ejected into the left ventricle. The left ventricle pumps the blood out to the entire body. (1-4.2) (FR7 p. 541; FRASA p. 58)

32.

B. In an infant (patient under 1 year of age), the preferred pulse to assess is the brachial pulse located between the bicep and tricep muscle on the inner aspect of the upper arm. The radial and carotid pulses are the most commonly assessed pulses in children (patient over 1 year of age) and adults. (1-4.2) (FR7 p. 157; FRASA p. 202)

33.

D. The site for gas exchange for cells throughout the body is in the capillaries. Arteries branch into aterioles that then lead into capillaries. Oxygen is passed from the capillary into the cell, and carbon dioxide is passed from the cell into the capillary. After the gas exchange, the blood leaves the capillary and enters a venule and then a vein. The veins transport the blood back to the right side of the heart and then to the lungs to pick up oxygen and dump off the carbon dioxide. (1-4.2) (FR7 p. 100; FRASA p. 58)

34.

C. The brain and spinal cord are components of the central nervous system. Peripheral nerves, which include sensory nerves and motor nerves, are not part of the central nervous system. (1-4.3) (FR7 p. 61; FRASA p. 59)

35.

A. In response to cold, the vessels in the skin constrict to shunt blood to the core of the body and to keep the warm blood out of the cold skin. In a hot environment, the vessels in the skin dilate to try to get the blood to the most peripheral parts of the body to allow the blood to cool. (1-4.4) (FR7 p. 159; FRASA p. 288)

36.

B. When lifting a patient, the back should be kept in a locked position that naturally forces an inward curve. (1-6.1) (FR7 p. 70; FRASA p. 75)

37.

C. Try to carry objects as close to your body as possible to prevent injury. Refrain from lifting and twisting at the same time. Keep your back locked in a natural position, not hyperextended. (1-6.2) (FR7 p. 70; FRASA p. 75)

38.

A. When possible and if medically appropriate, use a stair chair to move the patient down stairs. Typically, it is too difficult to maneuver the stretcher up and down steps. An extremity lift is used only to place the patient onto a device to move the patient. (1-6.4) (FR7 p. 83; FRASA p. 87)

39.

D. When carrying an object with one hand, you should avoid leaning too far to the opposite side. To prevent this unnatural position, keep your back in a locked position by keeping your abdominal muscles tight. When bending, you should bend at the hips, not at the waist. (1-6.5) (FR7 p. 70; FRASA pp. 75–77)

40.

C. The preferred method is to use a stair chair. A stair chair is used for the responsive patient who does not have a spinal injury. Using a stair chair will reduce the potential for lifting injuries. (1-6.6) (FR7 p. 83; FRASA p. 87)

41.

A. When performing the logroll technique, try to use your stronger shoulder muscles rather than your weaker back muscles. Support your body with your free hand, not your back muscles. When leaning toward the patient, try to lean at the hip, not the waist. (1-6.8) (FR7 p. 70; FRASA p. 75)

42.

A. Always push the object if possible. You are less apt to sustain an injury. (1-6.9) (FR7 p. 70; FRASA p. 75)

43.

B. You should use an emergency move only if there is an immediate danger to the patient or rescuer or to gain access to a more critically injured patient. Moving the first patient to gain access to a second patient who needs immediate life-saving treatment is correct. (1-6.11) (FR7 p. 71; FRASA pp. 78–79)

44.

B. The patient is displaying signs of possible tuberculosis (TB) infection, such as blood-tinged sputum, night sweats, and weight loss. Also, he is at higher risk for TB infection due to his HIV status. You should put on gloves and eye protection as a normal routine of body substance isolation protection and also put on a HEPA respirator or an N-95 mask. The HEPA respirator or N-95 mask will block out the very small TB bacteria and prevent transmission of the disease to you. If you are using a HEPA respirator that does not have an exhalation valve, you can place one on the patient also to reduce the incidence of respiratory droplet transmission. (*) (FR7 p. 44; FRASA p. 21)

45.

C. The patient has an altered mental status and is disoriented to time, place, and person. At this point, the patient is unable to make a rational decision and should be treated based on implied consent. If necessary, restrain the patient and provide emergency care. (*) (FR7 p. 23; FRASA p. 36)

2 Airway

module objectives

Questions in this module relate to D.O.T. objectives 2-1.1 to 2-1.18. There are also questions on enhanced topics, including bag-valve-mask ventilation and oxygen therapy.

DIRECTIONS Each of the questions or incomplete statements below is followed by suggested answers or completions. Select the **one answer** that is best in each case.

1. The epiglottis:
   A. closes shut over the trachea during inhalation.
   B. opens the esophagus during exhalation.
   C. blocks the opening of the trachea during swallowing.
   D. keeps air from entering the esophagus during ventilation.

2. The cricoid cartilage is located:
   A. in the superior portion of the larynx.
   B. lateral to the larynx.
   C. at the bifurcation of the trachea.
   D. inferior to the larynx.

3. Which range of respiratory rates indicates adequate breathing for a 6-year-old?
   A. 8–12 times a minute
   B. 12–20 times a minute
   C. 15–30 times a minute
   D. 25–50 times a minute

4. Which patient is breathing adequately?
   A. 8-year-old breathing 12 times a minute with a shallow tidal volume
   B. 3-month-old breathing 40 times a minute with abdominal movement
   C. 22-year-old breathing 26 times a minute with excessive accessory muscle use
   D. 61-year-old breathing 42 times a minute with a history of smoking

5. A sign of inadequate breathing in an infant is:
   A. a respiratory rate of 25–50 times a minute.
   B. a "seesaw" breathing motion.
   C. a regular respiratory pattern.
   D. an equal and full chest expansion.

6. If you are uncertain if a patient is breathing adequately after your assessment, you should:
   A. begin positive pressure ventilation.
   B. re-evaluate the patient's respiratory status.
   C. administer oxygen by nonrebreather mask.
   D. count the patient's respirations carefully over 1 minute.

7. A patient who exhibits excessive neck muscle use and retractions above the clavicles, above the sternum, between the ribs, and below the rib cage is most likely showing signs of:
   A. adequate breathing with tachypnea.
   B. bradypnea and hyperpnea.
   C. apnea and asystole.
   D. inadequate breathing.

8. You note a snoring sound upon assessment of the airway in an unresponsive patient who is found lying in bed. You should:
   A. place the patient on a nonrebreather mask at 15 liters per minute (lpm).
   B. tilt the head back and lift the chin forward.
   C. begin positive pressure ventilation with a pocket mask.
   D. assess to determine if a carotid pulse is present.

9. When performing a maneuver on an infant to open the airway, the head should be:
   A. hyperextended.
   B. kept in a neutral position or slightly extended.
   C. flexed forward.
   D. maximally extended with the shoulders elevated.

10. You are on the scene and find a 20-year-old female who has fallen from a second story window. You should open the airway by:
    A. head-tilt, chin-lift maneuver.
    B. head hypertension maneuver.
    C. lateral head lift maneuver.
    D. jaw-thrust maneuver.

11. What is the preferred method to open the airway of an infant who has not suffered any potential trauma or spinal injury?
    A. head-tilt, chin-lift with the head in a hyperextended position
    B. jaw-thrust maneuver with the head and neck in a neutral position
    C. head-tilt, chin-lift with the neck and head in a neutral position
    D. jaw-thrust maneuver with the neck in a hyperextended position

12. You are treating a 6-year-old who was struck by a car. The patient is unresponsive and has no gag reflex. You should open and maintain the airway by:
    A. jaw-thrust maneuver with head hyperextended.
    B. head-tilt, chin-lift, and oropharyngeal airway.
    C. head-tilt, chin-lift and a nasopharyngeal airway.
    D. jaw-thrust maneuver and an oropharyngeal airway.

13. When performing the jaw-thrust maneuver, the First Responder's elbows should:
    A. remain at least 2 inches above the surface on which the patient is lying.
    B. remain at least 6 inches above the surface on which the patient is lying.
    C. remain on the surface on which the patient is lying.
    D. be cradled securely on the rescuer's abdomen.

14. The jaw thrust maneuver opens the airway by:
    A. displacing the mandible forward.
    B. tilting the head back.
    C. tilting the head back and moving the jaw forward.
    D. retracting the lower lip.

15. What type of catheter is preferred for suctioning the oropharynx?
    A. soft
    B. rigid
    C. French
    D. bulb

16. After opening the mouth to assess the airway of a trauma patient during your initial assessment, you note a large amount of blood in the oropharynx. Your next immediate action should be to:
    A. suction the blood from the mouth.
    B. apply a nonrebreather mask and administer oxygen at 15 lpm.
    C. begin ventilating the patient with a pocket mask.
    D. assess the carotid or radial pulse.

17. Which of the following is the appropriate catheter and pressure for suctioning the nasal passage of an infant?
    A. soft catheter at 130–150 mmHg
    B. rigid catheter at 80–120 mmHg
    C. tonsil tip catheter at 130–150 mmHg
    D. French catheter at 80–20 mmHg

18. Select the correct statement pertaining to suction equipment or the technique:
    A. French or soft catheters are inserted beyond the base of the tongue in the infant.
    B. Suction should be limited to 15 seconds in the adult and 5 seconds in the infant.
    C. Suction should be applied before the catheter is inserted into the mouth.
    D. The convex side of the rigid catheter is placed against the tongue.

19. You arrive on the scene and find a 20-year-old male patient who has suffered a head injury from a fall. He has a large amount of blood and secretions seeping from the mouth. You attempt to open the mouth; however, the teeth are clenched almost completely shut. You decide to use a soft suction catheter to suction the oral cavity. How would you measure the soft suction catheter to determine the proper length?
    A. from the corner of the patient's mouth to the tip of the ear
    B. from the corner of the patient's mouth to the Adam's apple
    C. from the tip of the patient's nose to the tip of the patient's ear
    D. from the tip of the patient's nose to the patient's cricoid cartilage

20. What should the oxygen flow be set at, in lpm, when using a pocket face mask to ventilate a patient?
    A. 2 to 4
    B. 6 to 8
    C. 10 to 15
    D. greater than 15

21. When ventilating an infant with a pocket mask, the breaths should be delivered over _____ second(s).
    A. 1.0
    B. 1.5
    C. 2.0
    D. 2.5

22. You arrive on the scene and find a patient who fell off a scaffolding from about 30 feet. Upon assessment, you find sonorous (snoring) sounds, respirations are approximately 30 per minute and shallow, a radial pulse is absent, the carotid pulse is weak and rapid at about 130 bpm, and the skin is pale, cool, and clammy. You should immediately:
    A. immobilize the patient on a spine board.
    B. apply a cervical spinal immobilization collar.

C. stabilize the head and neck and apply a nonrebreather mask at 15 lpm and transport the patient.
D. perform a jaw-thrust maneuver with in-line stabilization and begin pocket mask ventilation.

23. When ventilating a patient while performing the jaw-thrust maneuver, it is necessary to:
    A. maintain a mask seal with one hand while tilting the forehead backwards.
    B. keep the mandible immobilized in a neutral position.
    C. hold a mask seal while lifting the mandible forward.
    D. flex the neck forward and push the mandible backwards.

24. The pocket-mask device without an oxygen source will deliver what percentage oxygen to the patient?
    A. 17 percent
    B. 21 percent
    C. 35 percent
    D. 100 percent

25. Which statement is true pertaining to the bag-valve-mask (BVM) device?
    A. The BVM generates a higher tidal volume than mouth to mask.
    B. The BVM is difficult to use and fatiguing to the operator.
    C. A non-disabling pop-off valve is a preferred feature on the BVM.
    D. Oropharyngeal airways are contraindicated when using the BVM.

26. You are preparing to ventilate a patient with the pocket mask. Choose the correct sequence for mask placement procedure.
    A. Place the narrow part of the mask over the bridge of the nose and the wider part over the cleft of the chin at the same time.
    B. Place the wider part of the mask over the cleft of the chin; then place the narrow part over the bridge of the nose.
    C. Place the narrow part of the mask over the cleft of the chin and then the wider part over the bridge of the nose.
    D. Place the narrow part of the mask over the bridge of the nose and then the wider part over the cleft of the chin.

27. When ventilating an adult with a pocket mask device connected to supplemental oxygen at a flow of 15 lpm, the breaths should be delivered over _____ second(s).
    A. 1.0
    B. 2.0
    C. 2.5
    D. 3.0

28. Ventilation of a patient with a BVM device is best performed by a minimum of _____ rescuers.
    A. one
    B. two
    C. three
    D. four

29. All of the following are indications that you are ventilating your patient adequately **except:**
    A. the chest rises and falls with each ventilation.
    B. the heart rate slows from 130 bpm to 80 bpm in an adult patient.
    C. the movement of the abdomen increases with each ventilation.
    D. the skin color begins to return to normal.

30. You arrive on the scene and find a 7-year-old patient who was pulled from a pond after being submerged for 10 minutes. The patient has a radial pulse of 92 bpm and is being ventilated by another First Responder by mouth-to-mask ventilation with supplemental oxygen connected to the device and flowing at a rate of 15 lpm. Ventilations are being provided at a rate of 12 per minute. The cyanosis persists after the initiation of ventilation. You should immediately:
    A. increase the ventilation rate to 20 per minute.
    B. decrease the oxygen liter flow from 15 lpm to 10 lpm.
    C. switch to mouth-to-mouth ventilation.
    D. begin chest compression.

31. A technique to determine if you are ventilating the patient effectively is to:
    A. observe the chest rise while squeezing the bag.
    B. listen for air sounds while squeezing the bag.
    C. feel the bag deflate when applying pressure.
    D. watch the patient's cheeks flare when ventilating.

32. Which of the following is likely to cause the abdomen to become distended while ventilating with a pocket mask?
    A. setting the oxygen supply regulator at 15 lpm
    B. allowing for passive exhalation after each ventilation
    C. using a nasopharyngeal airway
    D. ventilating to hard and too fast

33. What is the rate of ventilation for a child when ventilating with a mouth-to-barrier device?
    A. 12 to 20 ventilations per minute
    B. 12 to 15 ventilations per minute
    C. 10 to 12 ventilations per minute
    D. 6 to 7 ventilations per minute

34. You are attempting to ventilate a patient with a pocket mask device. The patient's chest does not rise. You should:
    A. increase the oxygen flow from 10 lpm to 15 lpm.
    B. deliver very quick forceful ventilations.
    C. re-evaluate the head position and the mask seal.
    D. begin chest compressions and continue ventilation.

35. When ventilating a patient with a pocket mask, the amount of volume of the ventilation delivered should be guided by:
    A. resistance felt in the airway.
    B. the sound of air escaping from the nose and mouth.
    C. the chest rise with each ventilation.
    D. a snoring sound when each ventilation is delivered.

36. When performing mouth-to-mouth ventilation with no supplemental oxygen, you should:
    A. reduce the rate of ventilation to 8 per minute.
    B. deliver the ventilation more forcefully over less than 1 second.
    C. deliver an estimated ventilation volume of 10 ml/kg.
    D. increase your rate of ventilation since supplemental oxygen is not used.

37. While performing mouth-to-stoma ventilation, you note minimal chest rise and air escaping from the mouth and nose with each ventilation. You should:
    A. pinch the nose and close the mouth and continue ventilation through the stoma.
    B. secure a mask seal over the nose and mouth, occlude the stoma, and continue ventilating the patient.
    C. apply a nonrebreather over the nose and mouth and administer 15 lpm of oxygen.
    D. insert a nasopharyngeal airway in the stoma and ventilate with a pediatric pocket mask.

38. What should you do if resistance is felt during the insertion of the nasopharyngeal airway?
    A. use greater force to continue the insertion of the airway device
    B. quickly remove the device and attempt to insert a larger diameter airway
    C. immediately suction the nasopharynx using a soft suction catheter
    D. twist and turn the device as you continue to insert the airway

39. You determine the proper size of an oropharyngeal airway by:
    A. measuring from the tip of the nose to the tip of the earlobe.
    B. measuring from the corner of the mouth to the tip of the earlobe.
    C. choosing the same length airway as the length of the index finger.
    D. using the size formula (16 + the patient's age in years) ÷ 4.

40. Which of the following statements pertaining to the oropharyngeal airway is **not** correct?
    A. The oropharyngeal airway protects the airway from aspiration of secretions and vomitus.
    B. The patient's mental status is a primary consideration when determining if the oropharyngeal airway can be inserted.
    C. An oropharyngeal airway that is too long can cause a completely obstructed airway.
    D. The oropharyngeal airway is sized by measuring from the corner of the mouth to the angle of the jaw.

41. The oropharyngeal airway is contraindicated in which of the following patients?
    A. trauma patient who responds to verbal stimuli
    B. cancer patient in cardiac arrest
    C. unresponsive diabetic patient
    D. stroke patient without a gag reflex

42. Prior to insertion, a nasopharyngeal airway should be lubricated with:

    A. a water-soluble lubricant.

    B. the patient's oral secretions.

    C. a petroleum-based lubricant.

    D. sterile saline or sterile water.

43. To determine the proper length of a nasopharyngeal airway, measure from the patient's:

    A. corner of the edge of the mouth to the tip of the nose.

    B. corner of the edge of the mouth to the tip of the earlobe.

    C. bridge of the nose to the tip of the chin.

    D. tip of the nose to the tip of the earlobe.

44. A properly sized nasopharyngeal airway should:

    A. fit snugly in the nostril and extend 2 inches beyond the tip of the nose.

    B. fit loosely in the nostril and extend 2 inches beyond the base of the tongue.

    C. be seated firmly with the flange against the nostril.

    D. blanch the skin of the nostril, insuring proper diameter.

45. You arrive on the scene and find a 6-month-old who is thrashing about, making an effort to breathe, but is not moving any air. You determine that the patient is suffering from an airway obstruction. You should immediately:

    A. perform five abdominal thrusts.

    B. perform five back slaps then five chest thrusts.

    C. open the mouth and perform a finger sweep.

    D. suction the mouth using a soft suction catheter.

46. Abdominal thrusts are performed in an attempt to relieve an airway obstruction in:

    A. infants, children, and adults.

    B. infants and children.

    C. children and adults.

    D. adults only.

SCENARIO

Questions 47–49 refer to the following scenario:

You arrive on the scene and find an unresponsive 10-year-old patient lying face-down on the couch in the living room of a residence. After ensuring the scene is safe, you place the patient in a supine position, open the airway, and check for breathing. There is no air movement and the chest is not rising. You attempt to ventilate the patient but are unable to.

47. What would be your next immediate action?

    A. reposition the head and jaw and attempt to ventilate again

    B. perform a finger sweep followed by another attempt to ventilate

    C. perform five abdominal thrusts and inspect the airway

    D. perform five back slaps and five chest thrusts followed by a finger sweep

48. Your previous management was not successful. You should then immediately:

    A. perform a blind finger sweep

    B. perform five abdominal thrusts

    C. begin chest compressions and ventilations

    D. perform five back slaps and five chest thrusts.

49. The steps of CPR should continue for a foreign body airway obstruction with the following step added:

    A. perform a tongue-jaw lift and inspect inside the mouth before each ventilation

    B. perform a finger sweep

    C. attempt to ventilate with 3 breaths instead of 2 after each set of chest compressions

    D. perform five abdominal thrusts.

SCENARIO

Questions 50–54 refer to the following scenario:

You arrive on the scene at the local restaurant and find a 56-year-old male patient who appears to be in severe respiratory distress. He is sitting at a dining table and leaning forward, coughing forcefully, and grasping at his throat. He is pale and diaphoretic. His wife states he was joking and laughing and suddenly started coughing and having a hard time breathing.

50. What do you suspect the patient is suffering from?
   A. a heart attack
   B. a complete airway obstruction
   C. a severe allergic reaction
   D. a partial (mild) airway obstruction

51. What is your first immediate action to manage this patient?
   A. perform five abdominal thrusts and reassess the airway
   B. place the patient in a supine position and perform five chest thrusts
   C. instruct the patient to continue to cough forcefully
   D. attempt to insert an oropharyngeal airway

52. You suddenly note the patient becomes much more aggressive and begins flailing his arms. The patient quits coughing. You do not note any air movement coming from the mouth or nose and you do not see the patient's chest rise with each attempt to breathe. You should immediately:
   A. place the patient on the ground and assess his airway.
   B. move behind the patient and perform abdominal thrusts.
   C. provide five back slaps and then five chest thrusts.
   D. place your fingers in the patient's mouth and attempt to retrieve the obstruction.

53. The patient suddenly becomes unresponsive and slumps forward. You place him in a supine position on the floor. Your next immediate action should be to:
   A. open the airway performing a tongue-jaw lift and begin ventilations and chest compressions.
   B. perform five abdominal thrusts and reassess the airway.
   C. insert an oropharyngeal or nasopharyngeal airway and attempt to ventilate.
   D. perform five chest thrusts and then five abdominal thrusts.

54. Once you have completed the above, you should next immediately:
   A. insert an oropharyngeal airway.
   B. look into patient's airway, remove object if visible, and attempt to ventilate.
   C. perform five abdominal thrusts.
   D. apply a nonrebreather mask at 15 lpm.

SCENARIO

Questions 55–58 refer to the following scenario:

You and your partner are enjoying a well-deserved break when you are dispatched to 8356 64th Avenue for a patient complaining of shortness of breath. While en route, you both take body substance isolation precautions. Upon arrival, you find the scene is safe. You both enter the house to find a 35-year-old female walking around the house complaining, "I can't breathe." You have the patient sit down, and you perform an initial assessment. The patient is breathing 20 times per minute with adequate chest rise. Her heart rate is 102 bpm and her skin is pale, cool, and clammy. You ask the patient if she has been prescribed a metered dose inhaler (MDI). She states, "My puffer is on the nightstand."

55. You determine the patient is breathing _____ and _____.
   A. inadequately, perform the Heimlich maneuver
   B. inadequately, provide positive pressure ventilation
   C. adequately, continue with the assessment
   D. adequately, insert a nasopharyngeal airway

56. The patient states she has taken six puffs on her inhaler over the last 10 minutes prior to your arrival. Which of the following side effects would you expect the patient to experience as a result of taking the drug?

    A. bradycardia and blurred vision

    B. hypertension and salivation

    C. tachycardia and nervousness

    D. hypotension and sweating

57. Your partner notices that the patient is breathing faster and with increased effort. The patient's mental status has deteriorated. She is also using her accessory muscles in her neck and chest to breathe. You quickly reassess the airway and hear and feel little air exchange. You should immediately:

    A. begin to provide positive pressure ventilation with a pocket mask or bag-valve-mask device that is connected to oxygen.

    B. administer high-flow oxygen by nonrebreather mask at 15 lpm.

    C. perform a blind finger sweep, insert a nasopharyngeal airway and apply a nonrebreather mask at 15 lpm.

    D. insert a soft suction catheter deep into the airway to remove any possible secretions.

58. When ventilating a patient with a pocket mask device, you should deliver a tidal volume of:

    A. 15 ml/kg over 2 seconds.

    B. 10 ml/kg over 1 second.

    C. 6 ml/kg over 1 second.

    D. 4 ml/kg over 1 second.

ENRICHMENT QUESTIONS

Oxygen Therapy

59. When applying a nonrebreather mask or nasal cannula to the patient:

    A. apply the device to the patient, attach the oxygen tubing to the flowmeter, and open the flowmeter to the desired lpm.

    B. attach the oxygen tubing to the flowmeter, open the flowmeter to the desired lpm, and apply the device to the patient.

    C. open the flowmeter and set the desired lpm, apply the device to the patient, attach the oxygen tubing to the flowmeter.

    D. attach the oxygen tubing to the flowmeter, apply the device to the patient, open the flowmeter and set the desired lpm.

60. An oxygen tank is full when the pressure gauge reads:

    A. 500 pounds per square inch (psi).

    B. 2,000 psi.

    C. 3,000 psi.

    D. 5,000 psi.

61. When using a nonrebreather mask, the oxygen flow regulator should be set at:

    A. 15 lpm.

    B. 10 lpm.

    C. 8 lpm.

    D. 6 lpm.

62. You are treating a 62-year-old with a history of chronic obstructive pulmonary disease (COPD). The patient states, "I can't breathe," and presents with signs of hypoxia. The preferred method for delivering oxygen to this patient is:

    A. nonrebreather mask with the oxygen set at 10 lpm.

    B. nonrebreather mask with the oxygen set at 15 lpm.

    C. nasal cannula device with the oxygen set at 8 lpm.

    D. nasal cannula device with the oxygen set at 6 lpm.

63. The preferred prehospital device for oxygen delivery to a patient who has adequate ventilation is the:

    A. nasal cannula.

    B. simple face mask.

    C. nonrebreather mask.

    D. Venturi mask.

64. The nonrebreather mask provides high concentrations of oxygen to a patient by:

    A. utilizing high oxygen liter flow rates.

    B. its rebreather mask design.

    C. connecting the oxygen supply tubing directly to the mask.

    D. allowing the patient to inhale the oxygen from an oxygen reservoir bag.

65. Your patient refuses to keep a nonrebreather mask on her face, even with extensive coaching. You should next:

    A. remove the nonrebreather mask.

    B. remove the nonrebreather mask and apply a nasal cannula.

    C. continue to coach the patient and hold the mask to her face.

    D. blow oxygen by her face with oxygen supply tubing.

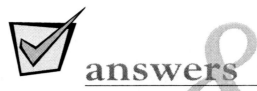

answers & rationales

Following each rationale, you will find a reference to the corresponding D.O.T. objective. A rationale marked with an asterisk denotes material supplemental to the First Responder curriculum. Also included after each rationale are references to where the question topic may be covered in Brady First Responder textbooks. **"FR7"** refers to *First Responder*, **7e** (Bergeron, Bizjak, Krause, Le Baudour). **"FRASA" refers to** *First Responder: A Skills Approach*, **7e** (Limmer, Karren, Hafen).

1.
C. The epiglottis is a cartilaginous flap of tissue that is responsible for closing shut over the opening of the trachea during swallowing. This prevents aspiration of food or other substances into the trachea and lungs. (2-1.1) (FR7 p. 100; FRASA p. 95)

2.
D. The cricoid cartilage, the only completely circumferential cartilaginous ring, is located inferior to the larynx. The cricoid ring is the landmark to perform the Sellick maneuver, also known as cricoid pressure. (2-1.1) (FRASA p. 95)

3.
C. The typical breathing rate range for children is 15–30 times each minute. The typical respiratory rate for the adult is 12–20 times each minute. The breathing rate of an infant is typically 25–50 times each minute. (2-1.2) (FR7 p. 100; FRASA p. 96)

4.
B. A 3-month-old breathing 40 times a minute with use of the abdomen is considered normal. An 8-year-old breathing 12 times a minute is slightly slow (average range is 15–30 times a minute). Low tidal volume means the depth of breathing is low (low air volume entering the lungs). A 42-year-old breathing 26 times a minute is fast (average range is 12–20 times a minute). Use of accessory muscles indicates increased effort to inflate the lungs. A 61-year-old breathing 42 times a minute is too fast, whether he or she is a smoker or not. (2-1.2) (FR7 p. 100; FRASA p. 96)

5.
B. A sign of inadequate breathing in an infant is a "seesaw" breathing motion. This results from the abdomen and chest moving in opposite directions during breathing. A respiratory rate of 25–50 in an infant is the average range. You should expect a reg-ular respiration with equal and full chest expansion. (2-1.2) (FR7 pp. 100–101; FRASA p. 103)

6.
A. You should begin positive pressure ventilation immediately. It is best to err on the side of safety and provide ventilation. (2-1.2) (FR7 p. 101; FRASA pp. 113–114)

7.
D. A patient with retractions above the clavicles, between the ribs and above the sternum, is most likely showing signs of inadequate breathing. Tachypnea is a rapid respiratory rate; bradypnea is a slow respiratory rate. Apnea is the absence of respiration. (2-1.2) (FR7 p. 101; FRASA p. 103)

8.
B. Snoring is an indication that the tongue is partially occluding the upper airway. Perform a head-tilt, chin-lift maneuver as a priority in establishing an airway. If the patient is suspected of having a possible spine injury, a jaw-thrust maneuver should be performed. (2-1.3) (FR7 pp. 101–102; FRASA pp. 98–99)

9.
B. Due to the underdeveloped structures of the upper airway in the infant, the head should be kept in a neutral position or slightly extended when performing a head-tilt, chin-lift maneuver. Hyperextending the head may actually cause the trachea to become occluded, causing an airway obstruction. (2-1.3) (FR7 pp. 108–109; FRASA pp. 99, 110, 140)

10.
D. The jaw-thrust maneuver does not require movement of the head or neck. This technique should be used when you suspect the patient may have a spine injury. The head-tilt, chin-lift requires the head to be moved, thus compromising the spine. (2-1.4) (FR7 pp. 102–103; FRASA p. 99)

11.

C. The preferred method for opening the airway of an infant without a suspected spinal injury is the head-tilt, chin-lift. It is important to remember that in the infant the head should be placed in a neutral position or slight sniffing position. If the head is overextended in the infant or child, the trachea may become obstructed. (2-1.3) (FR7 p. 109; FRASA pp. 99, 110)

12.

D. This patient may have a spinal injury; thus, you should open the airway by using the jaw-thrust maneuver. An oropharyngeal airway will aid in keeping the tongue away from the oropharynx, helping to maintain an open airway. (2-1.4) (FR7 p. 102; FRASA p. 99)

13.

C. When performing the jaw-thrust maneuver, the rescuer's elbows should be placed on the surface on which the patient is lying. This provides a solid surface to maintain spinal stabilization. (2-1.5) (FR7 p. 102; FRASA p. 99)

14.

A. The jaw-thrust maneuver opens the airway by displacing the mandible forward while maintaining the head in a neutral position. (2-1.5) (FR7 pp. 102–103; FRASA p. 99)

15.

B. A hard or rigid suction catheter—also known as a tonsil tip, tonsil sucker, or Yankauer—is the preferred catheter for performing oropharyngeal suctioning. The soft or French catheter is usually used to suction the nose, nasopharynx, or oropharynx. (2-1.7) (FR7 p. 130; FRASA pp. 126–127)

16.

A. Blood, vomitus, or other substances in the airway must be cleared immediately with suction. Failure to do so may lead to aspiration and severe hypoxia. Your suction equipment must always be ready for use. (2-1.6) (FR7 p. 129; FRASA pp. 126–127)

17.

D. The French or soft catheter is correct when suctioning the nasal passage of an infant. When suctioning the nasal passage of an infant, you should use low to medium suction (–80 to –120mmHg). A rigid (tonsil tip) catheter will cause injury to the soft tissue of the nasal passage. Suctioning at too high a suction (over 120 mmHg) may cause injury to the soft tissue of the nasal passage. (2-1.7) (FR7 p. 130; FRASA pp. 126–127)

18.

B. Suctioning longer than 15 seconds in the adult, 10 seconds in the child, and 5 seconds in the infant can cause hypoxia. The patient should be oxygenated before and immediately after suctioning. Inserting the catheter beyond the base of the tongue may injure soft tissue or stimulate nerves and cause a decrease in the heart rate. Suction should only be applied after the catheter is in place. The convex side of the rigid catheter is placed against the roof of the mouth, not the tongue. (2-1.7) (FR7 p. 130; FRASA pp. 126–127)

19.

A. The correct length of a French or soft catheter is determined by measuring from the patient's corner of the mouth to the tip of the ear when preparing to suction the oropharynx. If you are preparing to suction the nose or nasopharynx, you should measure from the tip of the patient's nose to the tip of the earlobe. (2-1.7) (FR7 p. 131; FRASA p. 127)

20.

D. When using a pocket face mask to ventilate a nonbreathing patient, the oxygen flow should be set at 15 lpm. (2-1.8) (FR7 p. 555)

21.

A. When ventilating an infant with the pocket mask, the breaths should be delivered over 1.0 second. The depth of ventilation should be just enough to allow for chest rise. (21.8) (FR7 p. 105; FRASA p. 109)

22.

D. The sonorous (snoring) sounds indicate a partially occluded airway. Thus, a manual maneuver must be performed to immediately open the airway. The jaw-thrust maneuver is the most appropriate due to the risk of possible spinal injury. Also, the patient's breathing is inadequate because of the poor tidal volume and excessively high rate. Therefore, it is necessary to immediately begin ventilation. Manual in-line stabilization should be performed at this point until the immediate life threats to the airway and breathing have been managed effectively. A cervical spinal immobilization collar should be applied during the focused history and physical exam. (2-1.4) (FR7 p. 102; FRASA p. 99)

23.

C. When performing the jaw-thrust maneuver, it is necessary to displace the mandible forward while keeping the head and neck in a neutral in-line position. This procedure is most commonly used for patients with suspected spinal injuries. (2-1.5) (FR7 pp. 102–103; FRASA p. 99)

24.

A. Using the pocket mask without an oxygen source will result in delivering only 17–18 percent oxygen, the amount found in the air we exhale. When used with an oxygen source at 10–15 lpm, you can achieve an approximately 40–50% oxygen concentration delivered to the patient. (2-1.8) (FR7 p. 547; FRASA p. 103)

25.

B. The BVM is difficult to use and fatiguing to the operator. If available, two First Responders should be used to ventilate a patient. One First Responder should hold the mask on the patient's face, while the other squeezes the bag. The BVM rarely is able to generate higher tidal volumes than the rescuer providing mouth to mask. A non-disabling pop-off valve is not preferred. A pop-off valve that is not disabled may lead to ineffective ventilation in some patients. The oropharyngeal airway will help to maintain an open airway in the unresponsive patient and is an appropriate adjunct to use when ventilating with the BVM. (2-1.8) (FR7 p. 548; FRASA p. 112)

26.

D. The proper sequence to place a mask on a patient's face is to first place the narrow part of the mask over the bridge of the nose, then lower the mask over the nose and mouth until the wider part meets the cleft of the chin. This sequence will aid in a better seal on the patient's face. If the mask does not cover the bridge of the nose and the cleft of the chin, you need to select a more appropriately sized mask. (2-1.8) (FR7 p. 105; FRASA p. 107)

27.

A. When ventilating an adult with a pocket mask, the breath should be delivered over 1 second. This slow ventilation prevents gastric distention. Observe for adequate chest rise and fall. (2-1.8) (FR7 p. 105; FRASA p. 109)

28.

B. Ventilation of a patient with a bag-valve-mask device is best performed by a minimum of two rescuers. One-rescuer BVM ventilation is discour-aged because it is difficult for one rescuer to maintain an effective seal and adequate volume of ventilation. (2-1.8) (FR7 p. 548; FRASA p. 112)

29.

C. An increase in abdominal movement or distention with each ventilation is an indication that air is being forced into the esophagus and stomach. This could potentially result in severe gastric distention that impedes ventilation and leads to aspiration. (2-1.8) (FR7 pp. 106–107; FRASA pp. 109, 111)

30.

A. The patient may not be adequately ventilated at a rate of 12 ventilations per minute. Infants and children can be ventilated at 12 to 20 ventilations per minute. Decreasing the oxygen liter flow will worsen the hypoxia state. The patient has an adequate pulse, and therefore chest compressions are not necessary. Mouth-to-mouth ventilation will not allow you to deliver supplemental oxygen and will cause cross-contamination, so it has no benefit in this situation. (2-1.9) (FR7 p. 109; FRASA p. 107–109)

31.

A. When ventilating a patient, watch for the chest to rise and fall. Often you will hear air sounds, but this could be air escaping around the mask. You should experience little resistance while ventilating. If it becomes more difficult to ventilate, consider repositioning the head, using an airway adjunct, or suspecting a tension pneumothorax. Often the cheeks will flare out with ventilations because they are flexible; however, this is not a sign that the lungs are being ventilated. (2-1.8) (FR7 p. 106; FRASA p. 109)

32.

D. Ventilating too fast with too high a tidal volume will force air into the esophagus and into the stomach, lessening the effectiveness of ventilation. To prevent air from entering the stomach, you should ventilate over 1 second and allow for passive exhalation. (2-1.8) (FR7 p. 112; FRASA p. 109, 111)

33.

A. When ventilating a child using a mouth to barrier device or pocket mask, he or she should be ventilated with 1 breath every 3 to 5 seconds, each breath delivered over 1 second. This would deliver 12 to 20 breaths per minutes. (2–1.8) (FR7 pp. 106–107; FRASA p. 109)

breaths per minutes. (2–1.8) (FR7 pp. 106–107; FRASA p. 109)

34.

C. Immediately assess the head and chin/jaw position or mask seal. If, after checking the head and chin/jaw position and mask seal, the chest still does not rise, an airway obstruction must be considered. Proceed with foreign body airway obstruction maneuvers. (2-1.8) (FR7 p. 107; FRASA p. 109)

35.

C. The proper volume of ventilation is determined by adequate chest rise with each ventilation. It doesn't matter if you are using a pocket mask or bag-valve-mask device. You should only be concerned with enough tidal volume to make the chest rise. (2-1.8) (FR7 pp. 106–107; FRASA p. 109)

36.

C. When providing positive pressure ventilation to a patient with a pocket mask device, deliver enough tidal volume to see chest rise. At 10 ml/kg the chest should rise adequately with each ventilation. (2-1.10) (FRASA p. 110)

37.

A. Air escaping from the nose and mouth while ventilating a patient through his stoma is an indication that the patient has a partial laryngectomy. You should pinch the nose and close the mouth and continue ventilation through the stoma. (2-1.10) (FR7 pp. 110–111; FRASA p. 110)

38.

D. A certain amount of resistance is expected when inserting a nasopharyngeal airway. If excessive resistance is encountered, remove the device and try the opposite nostril. Ensure that the airway is properly lubricated, and try gently rotating the airway from side to side. (2-1.12) (FR7 p. 129; FRASA p. 125)

39.

B. The proper method to size an oropharyngeal airway is to measure from the corner of the mouth to the tip of the earlobe or angle of the jaw. You can also measure from the center of the mouth to the bottom of the angle of the jaw. Sizing formulas are for tracheal tubes. (2-1.11) (FR7 pp. 126–127; FRASA pp. 123–124)

40.

A. The oropharyngeal airway does not protect the airway from aspiration of vomitus or secretions. Suction should always be available. You should only use the oropharyngeal airway on completely unresponsive patients. Failure to do so may result in the patient gagging and vomiting. Using an oropharyngeal airwar that is too long may force the epiglottis to close over the trachea, blocking the airway. (2-1.11) (FR7 p. 125; FRASA pp. 123–124)

41.

A. The oropharyngeal airway must only be used on completely unresponsive patients without a gag reflex. If the patient is semi-responsive, the patient may gag or vomit, causing further complications. (2-1.11) (FR7 p. 125; FRASA p. 123)

42.

A. Prior to insertion, a nasopharyngeal airway should be lubricated with a water-soluble lubricant. Never use a petroleum-based lubricant. (2-1.12) (FR7 p. 128; FRASA p. 124–125)

43.

D. To determine the proper length of a nasopharyngeal airway, measure from the tip of the nose to the tip of the earlobe. (2-1.12) (FR7 p. 128; FRASA p. 124)

44.

C. The presence of blanching at the nasal opening indicates that the nasopharyngeal airway is too large. Use a smaller-diameter airway. Blanching (when the nasal opening becomes white) is a result of blood being forced from the area from excessive pressure. The airway should be inserted until the flange is seated firmly on the nostril. (2-1.12) (FR7 p. 128; FRASA p. 124)

45.

B. Once you have definitely determined that the airway is obstructed because of an object and not infection or swelling, you should proceed with five back slaps and then five chest thrusts. You should continue until the infant becomes unresponsive or the obstruction is relieved. (2-1.15) (FR7 p. 114; FRASA pp. 139–140)

46.

C. Abdominal thrusts are performed on children and adults suffering from severe complete airway obstructions. Back slaps and chest thrusts are only performed on infants. (2-1.17) (FR7 pp. 114–115; FRASA pp. 138–140)

47.

A. If you are unable to ventilate, it may be because of a poorly positioned airway. You should immediately reposition the head and jaw and reattempt to ventilate. (2-1.17) (FR7 pp. 106, 114; FRASA p. 138)

48.

B. If repositioning of the airway did not relieve the obstruction, assume the patient is suffering from a foreign body airway obstruction. The next step is to begin CPR. Perform a tongue-jaw lift prior to each ventilation to look for the object. Finger sweeps are only to be done if you can visualize the object. (2-1.17) (FRASA p. 138)

49.

A. After performing each cycle of CPR (30:2), you must then perform a tongue-jaw lift and inspect inside the mouth. If the obstruction is seen, you should perform a finger sweep in an attempt to dislodge it. Do not perform a blind finger sweep. Afterwards, reposition the airway and attempt to ventilate. (2-1.17)

50.

D. Any patient who suffers a sudden onset of severe respiratory distress while eating should be suspected of having an airway obstruction. This patient is suffering a partial airway obstruction because he is still moving air. Evidence that the patient is still moving air is the coughing and stridor (high-pitched sounds) heard on inhalation and exhalation. (*) (FR7 p. 113; FRASA p. 135)

51.

C. Because the patient has a partial airway obstruction and is still moving air on his own, you should instruct the patient to continue to cough forcefully to try to cough out the obstruction. Have the patient assume a position of comfort, which is usually sitting straight up or leaning forward. Do not perform abdominal thrusts unless the patient has a complete airway obstruction. (2-1.13) (FR7 p. 114; FRASA p. 136)

52.

B. The patient has deteriorated to a complete airway obstruction; however, he remains responsive. You must move behind the patient, support his body, and apply abdominal thrusts. Continue to provide the abdominal thrusts until you have relieved the

obstruction, the patient becomes unresponsive, or other EMS units arrive on the scene. (2-1.16) (FRASA p. 137)

53.

A. If a responsive choking patient becomes unresponsive, you should immediately guide the patient to the floor, open the airway by performing a tongue-jaw lift, do a finger sweep only if you see the object, attempt to ventilate, and begin chest compressions. (2-1.16) (FRASA p. 138)

54.

B. Once you have performed a tongue-jaw thrust and finger sweep, and have attempted to ventilate, you should then begin chest compressions. (2-1.16) (FRASA pp. 100, 138)

55.

C. This patient's breathing status is adequate because the respiratory rate is normal, there is good chest rise, and there is good air volume being exchanged in the lungs. The patient was found walking around the house. Many patients with inadequate ventilation will assume a tripod position. You should continue with your assessment. (2-1.13) (FR7 pp. 100–101; FRASA pp. 102–103)

56.

C. The common side effects of a beta agonist drug are tachycardia, tremors, shakiness, nervousness, dry mouth, nausea, and vomiting. It is important to explain these common side effects to your patient prior to administering the drug. Explaining the common side effects will help to reduce the patient's stress and apprehension. (2-2.8) (FR7 p. 563)

57.

A. The patient's breathing has changed from adequate to inadequate. You should immediately provide positive pressure ventilation with a pocket mask or bag-valve-mask device and supplemental oxygen. Administering high-flow oxygen will not help this patient. You must facilitate delivery of oxygen to the lungs by using positive pressure ventilation (artificial ventilation or rescue breathing). This patient does not need deep suctioning. (2-1.2) (FR7 pp. 100–101; FRASA pp. 102–103)

58.

C. A tidal volume of 10 ml/kg over a 1-second period should be delivered when providing ventilation by pocket mask or bag-valve-mask device or without oxygen. The recommended liter flow to be used with the bag-valve-mask device and pocket mask is 15 lpm. (2-1.8)

59.

B. When administering oxygen to the patient, you should first set up the oxygen delivery system. Second, prepare and attach the oxygen delivery device to the flowmeter, set the desired lpm flow, then apply the device to the patient. Applying a nonrebreather to the patient without oxygen flow can reduce the patient's tidal volume and cause or increase hypoxia. (*) (FR7 p. 554; FRASA pp. 128–129)

60.

B. The best way to measure the volume in the oxygen tank, regardless of the size of tank, is the pressure gauge. A full tank has 2,000 psi of pressure. As the tank volume decreases, so does the pressure in the tank. (*) (FR7 p. 551; FRASA p. 128)

61.

A. When using a nonrebreather oxygen mask, the oxygen regulator must be set so that the reservoir on the mask remains inflated. Typically the oxygen flow required to keep the reservoir inflated is 15 lpm. (*) (FR7 p. 554; FRASA p. 129)

62.

B. In the prehospital setting, always provide high-flow oxygen to the COPD patient who is complaining of shortness of breath. The nasal cannula may not deliver enough oxygen to this patient; thus, the nonrebreather mask should be used. A nasal cannula set at 6 lpm will deliver only 44% oxygen. (*) (FR7 p. 553; FRASA pp. 128–129)

63.

C. The preferred prehospital device for oxygen delivery is the nonrebreather mask. It delivers about a 90–95% oxygen concentration to the patient with adequate ventilation. Adjust the flowmeter to prevent the nonrebreathing oxygen reservoir bag from completely collapsing when the patient inhales. This is usually 15 lpm. The nasal cannula is used only when a patient is not able to tolerate a nonrebreather mask. (*) (FR7 p. 554; FRASA p. 128)

64.

D. The nonrebreather mask provides high concentrations of oxygen primarily because the device contains an oxygen reservoir bag that collects 100% oxygen. The reservoir, in conjunction with high oxygen liter flow rates, allows the patient to inhale high concentrations of oxygen with each breath. (*) (FR7 p. 554; FRASA p. 129)

65.

B. If a patient is unable to tolerate a nonrebreather mask, you should first attempt to coach the patient. If that is not effective, a nasal cannula should be applied. If the patient cannot tolerate the nasal cannula, oxygen should be administered by the blow by technique. (*) (FR7 p. 553; FRASA p. 129)

3 Patient Assessment

module objectives

Questions in this module relate to D.O.T. objectives 3-1.1 to 3-1.21.

DIRECTIONS Each of the questions or incomplete statements below is followed by suggested answers or completions. Select the **one answer** that is best in each case.

1. Scene safety begins:
   A. when you have reached the patient's side.
   B. just prior to reaching the patient's side, so the patient will not be distracted when performing the initial assessment.
   C. as you are arriving at the scene and before even exiting your response vehicle.
   D. as you approach the scene once you have exited the response vehicle.

2. Which of the following characteristics of a scene or patient would make it the most dangerous and possibly pose the greatest hazard to the First Responder?
   A. a scene that attracts bystanders
   B. a patient who is just recovering from a seizure
   C. a scene that involves more than one patient so that triage is necessary
   D. a patient who may experience a sudden change in his or her behavior

3. While on the scene of an automobile crash, you find a small-diameter power line lying across the vehicle. Which of the following is correct regarding power lines?
   A. Power lines can safely be removed by using rubber gloves and a long pipe or pole.
   B. Consider all power lines to be energized until a power company representative tells you they are not.
   C. Power lines that are knocked down on the ground are grounded and pose no threat to the First Responder.
   D. Small-diameter power lines are low energy and can be safely removed without injury to you.

4. During the scene size-up, you identify a large, angry crowd in what appears to be a hostile environment. You should:
   A. approach the scene cautiously to calm down those at the scene.
   B. make brief contact with the patient to explain you will return, and leave the scene.
   C. drive past the scene, contact your communications center to dispatch police, and wait for the police to arrive.
   D. attempt to quickly gain access to the patient by announcing clearly that you are a First Responder and are there to help.

5. You are called, on a winter morning, to the house of a family of five who are complaining of flu-like symptoms with a rapid onset. The elderly grandmother and infant son are both very hard to arouse. You should suspect:
   A. a toxic environment.
   B. the influenza virus.
   C. hypothermia.
   D. poor nutritional state.

6. Which of the following scenes would **most** likely pose a threat to the First Responder?
   A. a crime scene where a patient has been shot
   B. a large crowd that has gathered at the scene
   C. a hypoxic patient who appears to be agitated
   D. a bar fight with a number of intoxicated patrons

7. Your major responsibility at a crime scene is to:
   A. provide emergency medical care.
   B. prevent unnecessary people from entering the scene.
   C. identify potential weapons and preserve evidence.
   D. console the family.

8. Immediately upon arriving at a crash scene, you should:
   A. determine the total number of patients.
   B. determine if downed wires are present.
   C. survey and assess the entire scene and its surrounding area.
   D. determine if any patients are ambulatory.

9. A patient who opens his eyes only when instructed to do so is considered to be:
   A. disoriented and responsive to verbal stimuli.
   B. responsive to verbal stimuli.
   C. alert and disoriented.
   D. alert and oriented.

10. All calls are typically categorized during the scene size-up and initial assessment as being:
    A. medical or obstetric.
    B. medical or trauma.
    C. trauma or cardiac.
    D. cardiac or respiratory.

11. Mechanism of injury includes all the following **except:**
    A. falls.
    B. myocardial infarction.
    C. motor vehicle crash.
    D. shootings.

12. You arrive on a scene and immediately determine that there are more patients than one EMS unit can manage. When should you call for additional assistance?
    A. before making patient contact
    B. after making patient contact
    C. after the police have arrived
    D. after a fire official has arrived

13. Determining the total number of patients at a scene is a part of the:
    A. initial assessment.
    B. focused history.
    C. patient assessment.
    D. scene size-up.

14. You arrive on the scene of a two-car motor vehicle crash. During your scene size-up, you find four patients who appear to have significant injuries. You should immediately:
    A. triage the patients.
    B. call for transport of the most critical patient.
    C. contact the hospital to notify it of the number of patients.
    D. call for additional EMS units.

15. Categorization of the patient as trauma is based primarily on what two factors?
    A. scene size-up and the patient's vital signs
    B. immediate assessment of the scene and the initial assessment
    C. assessment of the scene and the mechanism of injury
    D. immediate assessment of the scene and the patient's mental status

16. Which of the following is an example of non-purposeful movement to painful stimuli?
    A. The patient arches his or her back and flexes the arms toward the chest.
    B. The patient reaches up and grabs your hand in an attempt to remove pain.
    C. The patient makes attempts to move away from the painful stimulation.
    D. The patient moves his or her arm upwards and outwards in a sweeping motion toward the pain.

17. Which of the following would be a sign of a partially occluded airway?
    A. a patient who is able to give you his or her chief complaint with garbled speech
    B. an alert patient who has stridor on inhalation and is unable to speak
    C. a child who is crying vigorously and swallowing air
    D. an infant who is alert, breathing hard, and wheezing

18. You find a diabetic patient lying supine on the floor at the bottom of the stairs. Your first priority should be to:

    A. determine the mental status.

    B. provide manual in-line spinal stabilization.

    C. assess the patient's airway.

    D. assess the patient's breathing and pulse.

19. The most effective method to determine breathing status during the initial assessment is to:

    A. auscultate for breath sounds.

    B. inspect for retractions.

    C. apply a pulse oximeter.

    D. look, listen, and feel for air exchange.

20. After opening the airway by a head-tilt, chin-lift maneuver during your initial assessment of an elderly patient found lying supine in bed, you determine the patient is not breathing. You should immediately perform which of the following?

    A. provide positive pressure ventilation

    B. begin chest compressions and ventilation

    C. assess the circulation by checking a radial pulse

    D. begin a rapid head-to-toe assessment

21. You have been dispatched to the scene of a shooting. The local police have secured the scene. They direct you to the patient who is a male about 16 years of age. There is a large bloodstain on the left side of the patient's chest. The patient's eyes are closed, and he does not move as you approach. Your partner takes manual in-line stabilization and opens the airway using the jaw-thrust maneuver. Your next immediate action should be to:

    A. apply a gauze dressing to the chest wound.

    B. assess the breathing status.

    C. size and place a cervical collar on the patient.

    D. palpate the chest for signs of chest injury.

22. You are providing positive pressure ventilation by pocket mask with an oropharyngeal airway in place. Your partner has sealed a sucking chest wound with an occlusive dressing and controlled bleeding from the chest. You find that it is becoming increasingly difficult to ventilate the patient. You should immediately:

    A. listen for abnormal or absent breath sounds and ventilate with more force.

    B. recheck the patient's pulse and skin color.

    C. quickly release and then reseal the occlusive dressing, sealing the chest wound.

    D. recheck the liter flow of oxygen to the pocket mask.

23. During your physical exam you find a bullet wound in the occipital region of the patient's head. The patient's pupils are unequal, and a straw-colored fluid is draining from his right ear. You have inserted an oropharyngeal airway and you are ventilating with a bag-valve mask at 12 times per minute. You should:

    A. quickly remove the oropharyngeal airway.

    B. decrease the oxygen concentration provided.

    C. ventilate the patient at 8–12 ventilations per minute.

    D. increase the ventilation rate to 20 ventilations per minute.

24. During the initial assessment, you determined the unresponsive infant has an obstructed airway from a foreign body. Your initial action should be to perform:

    A. five quick chest thrusts.

    B. five abdominal thrusts.

    C. a blind finger sweep.

    D. five rapid back blows.

25. You are called to the scene for a 6-month-old infant who is sick. When you arrive on the scene, you remove the infant, who looks ill, from the parent who is holding her to do your assessment. The infant allows you to remove her and doesn't cry or seem to be bothered. You would assume the infant's mental status is:
    A. alert and oriented since the infant is not crying.
    B. decreased because the infant is not responding appropriately.
    C. normal because an infant does not normally recognize a parent at 6 months.
    D. decreased since she appears to be ill.

26. When initially assessing the pulse in an adult, the _____ artery is palpated, whereas in an infant you will be palpating the _____ artery.
    A. carotid, brachial
    B. radial, brachial
    C. radial, femoral
    D. brachial, radial

27. You arrive on the scene and find a patient who fell from a tree. His pants are soaked with blood. You expose the injured area and find a large laceration with a steady flow of blood. You should immediately:
    A. press your gloved hand firmly over the wound.
    B. apply a tourniquet directly below the wound.
    C. place a pressure dressing over the wound site.
    D. apply digital pressure to the nearest proximal pressure point.

28. You would expect a patient who has lost a significant amount of blood to present with which of the following skin temperatures?
    A. warm
    B. normal
    C. extremely cold
    D. cool

29. Capillary refill is a most reliable sign in:
    A. adults.
    B. children over 8 years of age.
    C. children less than 6 years of age.
    D. newborns only.

30. When reconsidering the mechanism of injury in the physical exam, you should determine if:
    A. the further evaluation of the mechanism of injury met criteria to be considered significant.
    B. any hazards or potential hazards that could harm you or the patient were missed.
    C. specific injury to organs can be identified.
    D. the airway or breathing is compromised.

31. Significant mechanism of injury in the infant and child includes all the following **except:**
    A. falls greater than 10 feet.
    B. motor vehicle collisions of low speed.
    C. bicycle collisions.
    D. motor vehicle collision with the death of a passenger in the same compartment as the patient.

32. In what order would you conduct an assessment of a patient with a significant mechanism of injury?
    A. initial assessment, head-to-toe physical exam, SAMPLE history
    B. initial assessment, SAMPLE history, head-to-toe physical exam
    C. head-to-toe physical exam, SAMPLE history, initial assessment
    D. SAMPLE history, initial assessment, head-to-toe physical exam

33. You arrive at the scene of a motor vehicle crash with significant vehicle damage. You find the patient unrestrained in the front seat. Following the scene size-up, you should immediately:
    A. perform an initial assessment.
    B. perform a physical exam to the head, chest, and abdomen.

C. obtain a SAMPLE history.

D. perform an ongoing assessment.

34. The First Responder physical exam:

A. is a focused exam on a specific injury site.

B. is a quick head-to-toe exam.

C. begins with obtaining a SAMPLE history.

D. is conducted based on the injury and patient condition.

35. The decision to perform a head-to-toe physical exam or focused physical exam is based on the:

A. patient's heart rate.

B. SAMPLE history.

C. mechanism of injury and initial assessment findings.

D. findings in the ongoing assessment.

36. You performed a focused physical exam on a patient who suffered a leg injury from a fall. As you are waiting for the EMS unit to arrive, the patient suddenly becomes disoriented and repeatedly asks you what happened. You should:

A. contact medical control for orders for further emergency care.

B. conduct a focused exam to the patient's head.

C. obtain a SAMPLE history.

D. perform a head-to-toe physical exam.

37. A physical exam that is conducted to identify life-threatening injuries to the head, chest, abdomen, pelvis, or extremities in a trauma patient is:

A. a focused physical exam.

B. an ongoing assessment.

C. an initial assessment.

D. head-to-toe physical exam.

38. Upon performing your initial assessment, you find the patient complaining of severe pain to his ankle following a fall while playing basketball. When questioned, he cannot identify where he is. This patient requires:

A. a rapid assessment of his SAMPLE history.

B. a focused physical exam.

C. a rapid head-to-toe physical exam.

D. an initial assessment and rapid transport.

39. The mnemonic DOTS stands for:

A. deformities, oxygen depletion, tension, swelling.

B. distension, open injuries, tenderness, swelling.

C. deformities, open injuries, tenderness, swelling.

D. distention, open injuries, tenderness, sweating.

40. The First Responder physical exam is performed on an adult using a systematic approach, starting at the _____ and ending at the _____?

A. lower extremities, head

B. head, pelvis

C. head, posterior body

D. upper extremities, lower extremities

41. When assessing the head and face of a trauma patient during the physical exam, you should:

A. remove the head immobilization device to allow for better examination of the head.

B. firmly press on the skull, using the tips of your fingers to feel for depressions.

C. note any areas of deformity to the skull, face, and upper and lower jaw.

D. apply pressure to each eye, assessing for injury to the globe.

42. While assessing the chest during the physical exam, you find very minimal chest rise during inhalation. You should:
    A. complete the assessment followed by application of oxygen by nonrebreather mask.
    B. complete the assessment and then provide positive pressure ventilation.
    C. immediately administer oxygen by non-rebreather mask and then continue the assessment.
    D. immediately begin positive pressure ventilation and continue with the assessment.

43. When performing a head-to-toe physical exam, which of the following represents a critical finding that must be managed immediately?
    A. paradoxical chest wall movement
    B. deformity to the lower leg
    C. neck veins that are distended
    D. an open humerus fracture with the bone protruding from the skin

44. The rapid First Responder head-to-toe physical exam is performed to:
    A. prevent patient complaints.
    B. identify life-threatening injuries or conditions.
    C. recognize life threats to the airway and breathing.
    D. identify detailed information about the injury.

45. When assessing a medical patient, it is important to ask questions concerning the chief complaint to:
    A. further assess the history of the present illness.
    B. base all treatment of the patient on.
    C. determine if advanced life support (ALS) assistance is needed.
    D. determine the mechanism of injury.

46. Which of the following is a helpful tool used to collect information about the chief complaint?
    A. detailed physical exam
    B. DCAP-BTLS mnemonic
    C. AVPU mnemonic
    D. OPQRST mnemonic

47. The OPQRST is a mnemonic for:
    A. onset, pain, quantity, radiation, sensation, time.
    B. onset, provocation/palliation, quality, radiation, severity, time.
    C. onset, pain, quality, radiation, sensation, time.
    D. onset, provocation, quantity, radiation, sensation, time.

48. When asking the patient about provocation/palliation, you are trying to determine:
    A. what makes the pain better or worse.
    B. what started the pain.
    C. the approximate time the pain started.
    D. what the patient was doing when the symptoms were first noticed.

49. While assessing a patient's complaint you ask, "Does the pain move to the jaw or down the arms?" This question is assessing the:
    A. quality.
    B. radiation.
    C. provocation.
    D. severity.

50. When assessing the quality of a patient's chest pain, you would ask which of the following questions?
    A. What does the pain feel like?
    B. Where is the pain?
    C. What makes the pain worse?
    D. When and how did the pain begin?

51. The exam for the responsive medical patient is performed in what sequence?
   A. history, physical exam, ongoing assessment
   B. history, ongoing assessment, physical exam
   C. physical exam, ongoing assessment, history
   D. ongoing assessment, history, physical exam

52. The examination of the unresponsive medical patient is performed in which sequence?
   A. history, physical exam, ongoing assessment
   B. history, ongoing assessment, physical exam
   C. physical exam, history, ongoing assessment
   D. ongoing assessment, history, physical exam

53. Which of the following best describes a patient who is considered to be in a coma or comatose?
   A. a patient who is not oriented to person, place, or time
   B. a patient who does not respond to verbal stimuli
   C. a patient who does not respond to any painful stimuli
   D. a patient whose eyes do not open spontaneously without any command

54. When assessing the unresponsive medical patient:
   A. perform a complete detailed physical exam immediately upon arrival at the scene.
   B. inspect the scene for information about the nature of the illness.
   C. do not ask bystanders and family members questions regarding the incident.
   D. perform the initial assessment after the rapid head-to-toe physical exam.

55. Unequal pupils may indicate:
   A. carbon monoxide poisoning.
   B. head injury.
   C. severe hypoxia.
   D. heat emergency.

56. Your medical patient responds to painful stimulation with non-purposeful movement during the initial assessment. After the initial assessment, you should next perform a:
   A. focused physical exam of the eyes.
   B. SAMPLE history interview.
   C. detailed physical exam of the head only.
   D. rapid head-to-toe physical exam.

57. The unresponsive medical patient should be placed in which position?
   A. Trendelenburg position
   B. semi-Fowler's position
   C. prone position, legs extended
   D. left lateral recumbent position

58. You have just completed the initial assessment on a medical patient complaining of shortness of breath. You would next:
   A. perform a rapid head-to-toe physical exam.
   B. further evaluate the chief complaint.
   C. perform a focused physical exam of the head.
   D. assess the patient by performing a focused physical exam of the chest.

59. During your ongoing assessment of a head-injured patient, you would repeat the initial assessment for all the following reasons **except:**
   A. to determine if the patient's injuries have begun to worsen.
   B. to make sure you did not miss any injuries in the rapid trauma exam.
   C. to determine if treatment provided is beneficial.
   D. to determine if you need to provide a different treatment.

60. Your patient was struck on the head with a hammer and lost consciousness. How often should you repeat the ongoing assessment?

    A. every 5 minutes

    B. every 7 minutes

    C. every 10 minutes

    D. every 15 minutes

61. Your patient has an altered mental status of an unknown cause. You have inserted an oropharyngeal airway to maintain an open airway. While you continue with the initial assessment, you should assess all the following except:

    A. positioning of the airway.

    B. for vomitus in the airway.

    C. for abdominal tenderness.

    D. the respiratory effort.

62. What is a purpose of frequently repeating the ongoing assessment?

    A. so that the hospital will not have to perform as many assessments upon arrival

    B. so that you can be sure you did not miss any major injuries in the rapid head-to-toe assessment

    C. to ensure that the First Responder is not sued for malpractice for missing an injury

    D. to identify trends in the patient's condition and to ensure that the treatment is effective

63. When performing an ongoing assessment on a stable patient, you should repeat and record vital signs and assessment findings every:

    A. 5 minutes.

    B. 10 minutes.

    C. 15 minutes.

    D. 20 minutes.

64. While performing an ongoing assessment your patient—who was initially alert and talking—is no longer talking and has his eyes closed. You should reassess the mental status using which mnemonic?

    A. OPQRST

    B. AVPU

    C. GLASGOW

    D. SAMPLE

65. During the ongoing assessment, you note the patient's pulse rate has decreased and is a poor quality. You should suspect:

    A. a low blood sugar level (hypoglycemia).

    B. a head injury or severe hypoxia.

    C. a heat-related emergency.

    D. an allergic reaction (anaphylaxis).

66. Which of the following is **not** a basic reason for performing an ongoing assessment?

    A. to determine a diagnosis of the patient's condition

    B. to detect any changes in the patient's condition

    C. to change the emergency care as needed

    D. to locate and identify missed injuries and conditions

67. Why should you wait at least one second after you push the transmit button before you begin speaking into the radio?

    A. to eliminate static in the background

    B. so your battery will last longer

    C. to allow the radio to broadcast farther

    D. to allow the repeater time to open the channel and prevent cutting off the first part of the communication

68. After you are finished with your transmission you should:

    A. turn the radio off to save power.

    B. say "Over" and wait for confirmation from the other participant.

    C. say "Over" and turn your radio off to free the airwaves.

    D. none of the above.

69. Identify the correct sequence of components of the brief radio report to responding EMS units:

    1. patient age and sex
    2. circulation status
    3. chief complaint
    4. airway and breathing status
    5. mental status

    A. 1, 2, 3, 5, 4
    B. 1, 3, 2, 5, 4
    C. 1, 3, 5, 4, 2
    D. 1, 3, 5, 2, 4

70. Once you have received an online order from medical direction, you should:

    A. repeat the order back word for word.
    B. ask medical direction to repeat the order.
    C. repeat the order to dispatch.
    D. ask your partner to repeat the order to you.

71. Essential information that needs to be included in the hand-off report to the EMS crew is provided in the following order in your oral report:

    1. circulation status
    2. age and sex
    3. interventions provided
    4. chief complaint
    5. SAMPLE history
    6. responsiveness
    7. physical findings
    8. airway and breathing status

    A. 2, 4, 6, 8, 1, 7, 5, 3
    B. 6, 2, 3, 8, 1, 5, 4, 7
    C. 2, 8, 1, 6, 4, 5, 7, 3
    D. 7, 8, 6, 4, 3, 1, 2, 5

72. To improve communication with your patient, especially children and infants, you should:

    A. immediately establish that you are in charge and allow the patient to speak only to you.
    B. position yourself at the same level or lower than that of the patient.
    C. address all patients by their first name.
    D. remove any other family, toys, or distractions from the area directly around the patient.

73. Which of the following characteristics is **not** true when dealing with an older patient?

    A. Not all older patients have auditory deficits.
    B. Some older adults need more time to rationalize what you are saying.
    C. Allow enough time for the patient to respond to your questions.
    D. Elderly patients often overdramatize their complaint of pain.

74. Which of the following is an appropriate procedure when using the radio to communicate with other members of the EMS team?

    A. Push the press-to-talk (PTT) button and immediately begin speaking.
    B. Speak with your mouth at least 12 to 18 inches from the microphone.
    C. Give objective or relevant subjective information, and avoid offering a diagnosis.
    D. After receiving medical control orders, stop the transmission and initiate treatment.

75. Medical direction insists that you perform a procedure outside of your scope of practice. You should:

    A. question the order.
    B. follow the order.
    C. call your supervisor.
    D. disregard the order.

SCENARIO

Questions 76–78 refer to the following scenario:

You and your partner Emil are dispatched to a call for a fight at 69 Over Street. Dispatch advises that the scene is secured by police, and they are requesting you to expedite your response. Upon your arrival, you are met by a police officer who states an elderly man named Carl Luis has been shot in the chest. As you approach the patient you quickly gain the impression that he is severely injured. You see blood escaping freely from a penetrating wound to the upper right chest. The patient is breathing approximately 20 times a minute.

76. As you proceed with the initial assessment, your first action should be to:

    A. assess mental status using AVPU.

    B. assess airway, breathing, and circulation.

    C. perform a focused history and physical.

    D. place your gloved hand over the chest wound.

77. The next action performed as part of the initial assessment of this patient is to:

    A. open the airway using the head-tilt chin-lift.

    B. assess mental status using the mnemonic AVPU.

    C. obtain a SAMPLE history and a detailed exam.

    D. establish manual in-line stabilization of the spine.

78. Relating to the mechanism of injury of this patient, which physical exam should you perform?

    A. focused physical exam

    B. rapid head-to-toe physical exam

    C. detailed physical of the chest

    D. concentrated trauma assessment

79. You are returning to quarters and stop by a convenience store to purchase a soft drink. A gentleman approaches and asks what was going on across the street from his house a few minutes ago. He identifies himself as the neighbor of the patient you just transported. How should you respond to his request?

    A. Tell him exactly what happened, but don't use any names.

    B. Tell him only if he promises not to tell where he got the information.

    C. Tell him this is "Off the record" and then relay the information.

    D. Tell him you are not allowed to divulge such information.

80. You arrive on the scene and find a 27-year-old man in the bathroom of his home. During your initial assessment, you determine he is not alert. The next immediate action you should take is to:

    A. open the airway by using a jaw-thrust maneuver.

    B. ask him to open his eyes or talk to you.

    C. insert an oropharyngeal airway.

    D. check for a radial pulse and skin color, temperature, and condition.

81. You arrive on the scene and find a young male construction worker who was crushed under a wall that collapsed on top of him. You determine the scene is safe and approach the patient. He is severely cyanotic and appears not to be breathing. Blood is spurting out of his cut pant leg. Your next immediate action should be to:

    A. begin positive pressure ventilation with supplemental oxygen.

    B. expose and apply direct pressure to the bleeding leg wound.

    C. assess the radial pulse and skin for perfusion status.

    D. take manual in-line stabilization and apply a nonrebreather mask.

82. You arrive on the scene and find a 30-year-old male patient with a gunshot wound to the chest. During your general impression you note blood in the mouth, severe cyanosis to the face and neck, and no chest wall movement. You should immediately:
    A. suction the airway and occlude the gunshot wound to the chest.
    B. expose the patient and check for other serious gunshot wounds.
    C. begin ventilation and place your gloved hand over the wound.
    D. occlude the open wound and apply a nonrebreather mask at 15 lpm.

83. You are assessing a 40-year-old male patient who crashed his motorcycle. He complains of pain to his right leg. You suspect the tibia and fibula are fractured. Which of the following would be the best indicator of a suspected fracture?
    A. crepitation
    B. pain
    C. ecchymosis
    D. edema

84. Which of the following provides the least accurate information when assessing circulation in the adult patient?
    A. capillary refill
    B. skin color
    C. skin condition
    D. peripheral pulse

85. While conducting your general impression, which of the following would cause you to believe the patient is having a difficult time breathing (dyspneic)?
    A. The patient is gasping for air while crying loudly.
    B. The patient is lying supine on the couch while explaining how he feels.
    C. The patient says a few words and takes a breath.
    D. The patient is on home oxygen at 2 lpm.

86. You arrive on the scene of an auto crash and find a 23-year-old woman who was the driver of the vehicle. During the initial assessment you find cyanosis to the face and neck, a large depression with moderate bleeding to the left temporal region, a respiratory rate of 12/minute with shallow breathing, and weak peripheral pulses. You should immediately:
    A. apply direct pressure to the head injury and apply oxygen.
    B. perform a jaw-thrust and begin ventilation.
    C. take a blood pressure and apply a pulse oximeter to determine the blood oxygen concentration.
    D. dress the wound to the head and then begin ventilation.

87. A 25-year-old female patient was thrown off her horse. She is responsive and complains of pain to her head. Following the initial assessment you should:
    A. conduct a focused physical exam of the head.
    B. have the patient drive herself to the hospital.
    C. conduct a detailed exam of the head.
    D. conduct a head-to-toe physical exam.

88. You arrive on the scene and find a 28-year-old female who fell 20 feet while roofing a house. As you exit the first-response vehicle, she appears to be unresponsive. You notice a large pool of blood around her left thigh. There is blood draining from the mouth and nose. Your first priority is to:
    A. suction the airway and begin ventilation.
    B. look for safety hazards before approaching the patient.
    C. expose the left thigh and find any possible major bleeding.
    D. open her airway using a jaw-thrust and apply a nonrebreather mask at 15 lpm.

89. You arrive on the scene and find a 10-year-old male patient who was struck by a car while riding his bike. He is unresponsive to painful stimuli. You have opened the airway with a jaw-thrust and find the respirations to be 20/minute and shallow. His radial pulse is barely palpable. You should immediately:

    A. apply a nonrebreather at 15 lpm.

    B. begin chest compressions.

    C. begin pocket mask ventilation.

    D. apply a cervical spinal immobilization collar.

90. A 62-year-old female patient whom you find sitting in her recliner at home is complaining of severe abdominal pain as you walk in the door. As you approach the patient, she states that her "belly is real sore and aching bad." Your next action in assessing the patient is to:

    A. assess the radial pulse and skin color, temperature, and condition.

    B. open the airway and assess the breathing status.

    C. begin ventilation and connect supplemental oxygen.

    D. conduct a rapid head-to-toe physical exam.

91. You arrive on the scene and find an 8-year-old boy at the local gym who was knocked out while playing basketball. Following your assessment, you suspect he has a head injury. You should immediately:

    A. call for transport without treatment due to the lack of parental consent.

    B. initiate emergency care and contact the EMS unit to provide an oral report.

    C. wait for the police to arrive before initiating treatment.

    D. contact the parents for consent to begin treatment.

92. You arrive on the scene and find a 23-year-old female patient who stepped on a piece of glass and lacerated her foot while walking through the front yard. She is sitting on the ground holding her foot as you approach her. She complains that her foot "hurts real bad" and is bleeding. Your next immediate action is to:

    A. assess the amount of bleeding to determine if it is uncontrolled and major.

    B. begin ventilation with a pocket mask device.

    C. immediately begin a rapid head-to-toe exam to assess for life-threatening injuries.

    D. perform a jaw-thrust maneuver and assess the breathing status.

93. Following the initial assessment of a medical patient complaining of chest pain, you determine that the patient is not oriented and is speaking inappropriately. The next step in your assessment is to:

    A. repeat the initial assessment.

    B. perform an ongoing assessment.

    C. conduct a focused physical exam.

    D. perform a rapid head-to-toe physical exam.

94. You arrive on the scene of an auto crash involving a frontal collision and find the patient seated in the front seat of the driver's side of the vehicle. You determine that the scene is safe and approach the patient. You should immediately:

    A. determine the mental status.

    B. open the airway using the jaw-thrust maneuver.

    C. establish manual in-line stabilization of the head and neck.

    D. assess the radial pulse and carotid pulses and the skin.

95. You arrive on the scene and find a 20-year-old male patient who was involved in an auto crash. Upon your assessment, you note the patient cannot tell you what date it is, where he is, or whom he is with. The patient refuses to let you examine him further and refuses any emergency care. You should:
   A. have the patient sign a refusal form and leave the scene.
   B. turn the patient over to the police on the scene and leave.
   C. begin to administer emergency care to the patient, using restraints if necessary.
   D. have the police transport the patient to the hospital in the police car.

96. Capillary refill would be most reliable and provide the most information on which of the following patients?
   A. a 3-year-old trauma patient who is trapped in a vehicle in 10° temperature
   B. an 8-year-old who is having an asthma attack
   C. a 30-year-old who was shot in the chest three times
   D. a 5-year-old who lacerated his femoral artery on broken glass and is bleeding profusely

97. Blood mixed with clear fluid coming from the ears in a patient who was struck in the head would most likely indicate:
   A. a fractured skull.
   B. a concussion.
   C. an injury to the ear canal.
   D. a lacerated meningeal artery.

98. You arrive on the scene and find a 74-year-old male patient who collapsed at home. As you approach the patient, you note his eyes are not open, you hear a loud gurgling noise, and it appears he is breathing at about 6 times per minute. You should immediately:
   A. assess the radial and then the carotid pulse.
   B. begin ventilation and assess his mental status.

   C. apply a nonrebreather mask and assess the blood pressure.
   D. apply suction to clear the airway and then begin ventilation.

99. The respiratory rate of an infant:
   A. is approximately the same rate as that of an adult.
   B. is usually slightly slower than that of an adult.
   C. is higher at birth and progressively decreases with age.
   D. is irregularly irregular.

100. You arrive on the scene and find a patient who is complaining of dizziness and nausea. You find the radial pulse is present and the skin is warm, moist, and flushed. You should next:
   A. determine the level of responsiveness.
   B. begin a rapid head-to-toe physical exam.
   C. gather a SAMPLE history.
   D. assess the patient's abdomen for tenderness and rigidity.

101. The skin is assessed during the initial assessment to determine the:
   A. level of hypoxia.
   B. number of circulating red blood cells.
   C. the perfusion status of the patient.
   D. need for oxygen therapy.

102. Which of the following is **not** considered a life-threatening injury?
   A. fractured ribs
   B. fracture to both femurs
   C. open wound to the posterior thorax
   D. unstable pelvis

SCENARIO

Questions 103 and 104 refer to the following scenario:

You arrive on the scene and find a 77-year-old male patient lying in bed. He does not respond to verbal stimuli. He is breathing at 22 times per minute with good tidal volume and his radial pulse is 78 bpm. The skin is warm, dry, and normal in color.

103. Your next immediate action for this patient is to:

A. apply a nonrebreather mask if available and begin a rapid head-to-toe physical exam.

B. establish manual in-line spinal stabilization and insert an oropharyngeal airway.

C. perform a physical exam on his head.

D. begin ventilation by pocket mask.

104. The skin of the patient most likely indicates:

A. hypovolemic shock.

B. inadequate delivery of hemoglobin to the cells.

C. good tissue perfusion.

D. hypoxia and hypercarbia.

105. The unresponsive medical patient should be placed in what position?

A. supine with head slightly elevated

B. Fowler's

C. left lateral recumbent

D. Trendelenburg

106. Which of the following is considered a symptom?

A. a swollen, deformed extremity

B. a heart rate of 110 bpm

C. neck muscle use while breathing

D. pain in the upper abdomen

SCENARIO

Questions 107 and 108 refer to the following scenario:

As you are pulling up to the scene of a construction accident you spot a patient lying prone on the ground next to a pile of rubble. It appears a building has collapsed.

107. Your immediate action is to:

A. take in-line spinal stabilization and logroll the patient onto his back.

B. assess the mental status and determine if he is responsive.

C. search for more than one patient and call for additional resources.

D. wait by the first-response vehicle until the engineer has indicated that the structure is safe to enter.

108. The next step in managing the patient is to:

A. roll the patient onto his side to check for responsiveness and for an open airway.

B. insert an oropharyngeal airway and begin positive pressure ventilation.

C. establish manual in-line spinal stabilization and logroll the patient into a supine position.

D. gather a SAMPLE history while your partner does the initial assessment.

109. You arrive on the scene and find a 16-year-old male patient lying on the living room floor in a fetal position (curled up with his knees drawn to his chest). His positioning would cause you to most likely suspect he is suffering from:

A. an asthma attack.

B. congestive heart failure.

C. appendicitis.

D. a migraine.

110. You arrive on the scene of a bar fight and find a male patient who is approximately 26 years of age who was struck several times in the face. The patient is hostile and not cooperating. He cannot remember his address or his last name and does not know where he is. He refuses to allow you to assess him or provide any emergency care. You should:

    A. have him sign a refusal form and leave the scene.

    B. explain the consequences of not allowing you to assess and treat him, document it on your report, and have the patient and a witness sign the refusal form.

    C. call for the police, restrain the patient, and conduct a rapid head-to-toe physical exam to identify any life-threatening injuries.

    D. have his friend who is at the bar with him drive him to the hospital as you follow close behind.

111. You arrive on the scene and find a 23-year-old pregnant patient trapped in her car that is on its roof following a broadside collision. Upon arrival at the scene, you should:

    A. gain access to the vehicle and take manual in-line spinal stabilization.

    B. immediately apply a nonrebreather mask at 15 lpm to the patient to try to protect the fetus.

    C. call for a second ambulance in case she goes into labor and delivers at the scene.

    D. wait until the fire department has stabilized the vehicle before gaining access to the patient.

112. During your First Responder physical exam of a patient who fell down the steps, you note that the unresponsive patient's left pupil is fixed and dilated. You would suspect the patient most likely:

    A. has suffered a brain injury.

    B. injured the eighth cranial nerve.

    C. has injured the eyeball during the fall.

    D. fractured the maxilla and mandible.

SCENARIO

Questions 165 and 166 refer to the following scenario:

You arrive on the scene and find a 34-year-old female patient who crashed her motorcycle. During your assessment, you note that the skin is pale, cool, and clammy; the abdomen is rigid and tender; and the radial pulse is weak and rapid.

113. Based on this information, you would suspect the patient is most likely suffering from which of the following?

    A. intra-abdominal bleeding

    B. a fibula fracture

    C. a pneumothorax

    D. bilateral femur fractures

114. The abdominal pain and tenderness in the patient is most likely due to:

    A. blood collecting around the femur.

    B. blood irritating the peritoneal lining of the abdomen.

    C. fecal material causing diaphragmatic irritation.

    D. the pleural lining collapse.

115. While you are collecting the SAMPLE history during the history and physical exam on a medical patient complaining of dyspnea, the patient states that he feels his breathing is much better when he sits straight up. This would be reported as an item addressing what component of the mnemonic OPQRST?

    A. severity

    B. provocation/palliation (alleviation)

    C. radiation

    D. quality

116. Pain upon palpation of the symphysis pubis most likely indicates:
    A. a bladder infection.
    B. a ruptured ovary.
    C. a pelvic fracture.
    D. intra-abdominal bleeding.

117. You are treating a 46-year-old male patient at the scene of an auto crash. He is complaining of pelvic pain and abdominal discomfort. An ongoing assessment should be conducted every:
    A. 30 minutes.
    B. 15 minutes.
    C. 5 minutes.
    D. 2 minutes.

118. You are conducting a focused physical exam on a patient complaining of chest pain. Which of the following assessments would **not** be included in your examination?
    A. inspection of the oral mucosa
    B. inspection of the chest
    C. inspection of the ears and nose
    D. assessment of the pedal pulses

119. You have just accompanied the EMS crew on a transport of a patient suspected of having a heart attack to the emergency department. Upon your arrival, you are greeted at the door by the ward clerk who instructs you to place the patient in room B. As you are transferring the patient over to the hospital bed, you receive a tone from your dispatcher for another emergency call. You should:
    A. immediately leave the emergency department and respond to the call.
    B. wait to notify the nurse or physician of the patient's condition prior to leaving.
    C. refuse to take the call until your prehospital report is completely done.
    D. instruct the ward clerk to pass the information about the patient to the physician.

120. Which of the following would **not** be considered a significant mechanism of injury?
    A. an auto crash with frontal impact
    B. a gunshot wound to the neck
    C. a deformed steering wheel in a rear-end collision
    D. a fall of less than two times the height of the patient

SCENARIO

Questions 121–123 refer to the following scenario:

You arrive on the scene and find a patient who fell off a balcony at a hard rock concert. He struck several people when he fell before being impaled on a broken piece of plastic. Upon your arrival at the scene, you note three people lying on the ground next to the patient.

121. As you enter the scene, what would be your immediate action?
    A. Perform an initial assessment on each patient to determine who is the most severely injured.
    B. Ask that the police remove all of the people at the concert before approaching the patient.
    C. Call for at least two additional ambulances to respond to the scene.
    D. Go right to the patient impaled on the plastic and begin your assessment.

122. You are now treating the patient impaled on the plastic. You take in-line spinal stabilization and note a large pool of blood around the left thigh where the clothing is soaked in blood. The patient is moaning and groaning in pain. You should immediately:
    A. apply a tourniquet to the leg to stop the bleeding.
    B. expose the extremity to assess for major bleeding.

C. check the radial pulse to determine if the patient is in shock.

D. assess the airway and breathing and apply a nonrebreather mask at 15 lpm if available.

123. Which of the following would be the **lowest** priority?

A. absent radial pulses with a weak and thready carotid pulse

B. pale, cool, clammy skin in a trauma patient

C. dizziness and weakness in a diabetic patient

D. open wound to the lateral chest at the fourth intercostal space

124. A 30-year-old female patient fell off of her bicycle. She was not wearing a helmet. During your physical exam, you notice discoloration to the mastoid process behind her left ear. This is most likely a sign of a(n):

A. infraorbital fracture.

B. basilar skull fracture.

C. fractured nose.

D. zygomatic arch injury.

125. You are treating a 2-year-old girl who has been vomiting and suffering diarrhea for the past 3 days. The best method to assess whether she has lost a significant amount of volume is by:

A. taking a systolic and diastolic blood pressure.

B. assessing the radial pulses and skin color, temperature, and condition.

C. determining the mental status and if she is oriented × 3.

D. inspecting the sclera for redness.

126. When conducting the initial assessment, you should always assume that the patient with an altered mental status:

A. has a head injury.

B. cannot maintain his or her own airway.

C. needs bag-valve-mask ventilation with supplemental oxygen.

D. will not have radial pulses.

127. You arrive at the scene of a bar fight and find a 25-year-old man who has been stabbed several times and is bleeding severely from a wound to the neck, which is spurting bright red blood. The dispatcher informs you that the assailant is still on the scene in the bathroom, cleaning blood off of his hands. You can hear the sirens of the police who are not yet on the scene. How would you proceed?

A. Try to keep the assailant calm and in the bathroom while you quickly apply direct pressure to the knife wound in the patient's neck.

B. Both you and your partner ask the assailant to put the knife down so that you can enter the bar and take care of the patient.

C. Remain in your vehicle until the police arrive on the scene and indicate it is safe to enter.

D. As soon as you see the police cars, quickly enter the scene and apply direct pressure to the wound, and drag the patient to safety.

128. An example of paradoxical motion of the chest is when:

A. a segment moves inward on exhalation.

B. a segment moves outward on exhalation.

C. a segment moves outward on inhalation.

D. a segment does not move with respiration.

129. Stridor is an indication of:

A. fluid or vomitus obstructing the upper airway.

B. bronchoconstriction and mucus obstructing the lower airway.

C. the tongue blocking the upper airway.

D. laryngeal edema partially occluding the upper airway.

130. You arrive at the scene of a fall and find a 42-year-old woman sitting on the ground next to a ladder. She says she only fell a couple of feet and twisted her ankle. She is complaining of a sharp stabbing pain in her ankle. Which component of the initial assessment must be assessed next in this patient?

    A. mental status

    B. airway

    C. breathing

    D. circulation

131. A 62-year-old female patient who has been working in her garden has hot, dry skin. This patient may be suffering from:

    A. a heart attack.

    B. heat exposure.

    C. shock.

    D. stroke.

132. You are assessing a 23-year-old female patient who is complaining of abdominal pain. While you are gathering your history, it is important to ask her which of the following questions?

    A. When was the last time you had intercourse?

    B. Have you ever smoked crack cocaine?

    C. Are you a drug user?

    D. When was your last period?

133. You are assessing a patient complaining of chest pain. You obtain a set of vital signs and find the following: BP 112/64, HR 112 bpm, and RR 16/minute. You should report that the patient has:

    A. a narrow pulse pressure.

    B. tachypnea.

    C. tachycardia.

    D. hypertension.

134. While assessing the trauma patient, you logroll the patient and find an open wound to the posterior thorax. You should immediately:

    A. increase the liter flow of oxygen to 15.

    B. begin BVM ventilation.

    C. assess the lower extremities for other wounds.

    D. apply an occlusive dressing.

135. The medical term for swelling is:

    A. erythema.

    B. edema.

    C. ecchymosis.

    D. contusion.

136. You arrive on the scene and find a patient who aspirated a large amount of vomitus. You would expect to find which of the following early in the assessment?

    A. pale, cool, clammy skin

    B. severe cyanosis

    C. constricted pupils

    D. high blood pressure

137. You arrive on the scene and find a patient who has fallen down the steps. As you approach the patient she states, "I am fine, but embarrassed. Just leave me alone and I'll be fine." You should immediately:

    A. take in-line spinal stabilization.

    B. open the airway and check inside the mouth.

    C. have her sign a refusal form.

    D. ask if it is okay to assess her to determine if she is injured.

138. A patient suffering an allergic reaction would most likely have:

    A. crackles.

    B. decreased breath sounds on one side.

    C. hives, itching, and wheezing.

    D. gurgling sounds in the upper airway.

139. Which of the following may be the best sign that an unresponsive patient may have suffered a seizure?

    A. a rapid radial pulse

    B. an increased systolic blood pressure

    C. poor capillary refill in the nail beds

    D. a lacerated tongue

140. An initial assessment must be conducted on:

    A. patients who present with an altered mental status only.

    B. all patients with either an illness or injury.

    C. those patients who would require an immediate intervention.

    D. patients when time and patient condition permits.

141. The purpose of the First Responder rapid head-to-toe physical exam is to:

    A. identify and manage life threats to the patient.

    B. locate all injuries to the patient.

    C. assess the airway, breathing, and circulatory status.

    D. identify injuries that will require surgical interventions.

142. Which of the following signs would indicate that the patient is having trouble breathing?

    A. The patient talks in a normal speech pattern.

    B. The patient is crying vigorously.

    C. The patient says a few words and gasps for a breath.

    D. The patient complains his throat feels as though it is closing.

143. You are treating a 28-year-old female who fell 20 feet while roofing a house. After determining she is unresponsive, you would immediately:

    A. open her airway using a head-tilt chin-lift maneuver.

    B. apply manual in-line spine stabilization and open her airway.

    C. start high concentration oxygen using a nonrebreather mask.

    D. open her airway and start pocket mask ventilation.

144. You are treating a 78-year-old female patient who was found at home on the living room floor by her daughter. She is unresponsive to painful stimuli. Her respirations are 15 per minute with very minimal chest wall movement. What should you do first?

    A. Apply a nonrebreather mask at 15 lpm and assess the pulse.

    B. Provide two ventilations and reassess the mental status.

    C. Immediately move the patient outside to wait for the ambulance to begin transport.

    D. Insert an oropharyngeal airway and begin ventilation.

145. During palpation of the abdomen in the First Responder physical exam, the patient makes a facial grimace and draws his knees upward. You would note this as abdominal:

    A. rigidity.

    B. tenderness.

    C. guarding.

    D. pain.

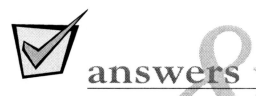

answers & rationales

Following each rationale, you will find a reference to the corresponding D.O.T. objective. A rationale marked with an asterisk denotes material supplemental to the First Responder curriculum. Also included after each rationale are references to where the question topic may be covered in Brady First Responder textbooks. **"FR7" refers to *First Responder*, 7e** (Bergeron, Bizjak, Krause, Le Baudour). **"FRASA" refers to *First Responder: A Skills Approach*, 7e** (Limmer, Karren, Hafen).

1.

C. The scene survey should begin as you are pulling up to the scene. You should be identifying potential hazards (fire, downed power lines, gas leaks) and also looking for clues to identify an unsafe scene (all the lights off in the house, general atmosphere of the scene, listening for arguing or fighting) before leaving the confines of the ambulance. (3-1.1) (FR7 p. 147; FRASA p. 179)

2.

D. A scene that involves a patient who may experience a sudden change in behavior poses the greatest risk to the First Responder. The patient may be intoxicated, under the influence of drugs, or suffering from a behavioral disorder. Unless bystanders become hostile, they do not pose a threat. A post ictal patient is typically confused and severely exhausted and rarely a threat. (3-1.2) (FR7 p. 270; FRASA p. 181–182)

3.

B. All power lines are considered energized until a power company representative arrives on the scene and advises you they are not. Downed power lines pose a serious threat to rescuers and the public. You should advise the patients to remain inside the vehicle until you can safely remove them. Never try to move power lines. Power lines that are on the ground can energize the area around them. Keep a safe distance away. (3-1.2) (FR7 pp. 147, 503; FRASA p. 393)

4.

C. If at any time you feel the scene is not safe, you have a few options: 1) if possible, make the scene safe; 2) retreat quickly and contact the necessary resources to make the scene safe; or 3) do not enter an unsafe scene. There is no reason to assess this scene further. You have identified it as a hostile scene; therefore, you should not attempt to enter it. Since there is a large crowd, you cannot possibly make the scene safe. Do not make contact with bystanders or the patient until the scene is secured by the police. (3-1.3) (FR7 p. 50; FRASA p. 181–182)

5.

A. In a closed environment like a house, when more than one patient complains of the same symptoms, you should suspect a toxic environment such as carbon monoxide poisoning. Clues that lead you to suspect a toxic environment in this situation include winter morning (high furnace use), inside the house (enclosed space with little ventilation), more than one patient with the same symptoms. In addition, with carbon monoxide poisoning, elderly persons, young children, and pets are affected first, presenting with more severe signs and symptoms. The elderly are affected earlier due to pre-existing medical conditions and deteriorated physiologic states. Young children and pets have a much higher metabolism than adults; thus, carbon monoxide affects the cells at a much higher rate. (3-1.2) (FR7 p. 148; FRASA p. 182)

6.

D. Of the scenes listed, the most dangerous is the barroom. Scenes in which First Responders and EMS personnel are most often injured are where the patient has a tendency to change his or her behavior abruptly. These are patients who are typically under the influence of drugs or alcohol or those suffering from mental instability. Typically, the perpetrator is long gone prior to the arrival of First Responders, the EMS crew, or the police at the scene of a shooting or stabbing. It is very unlikely that the perpetrator will stay on the scene. Regardless, First Responders should contact police and wait until they have cleared the scene of any safety hazards prior to entering. A large crowd is not a threat unless it appears to be hostile or agitated. (3-1.3) (FR7 p. 50; FRASA pp. 181–182)

7.

A. Your first and foremost responsibility at the crime scene is to provide emergency medical care. If possible, prevent destruction of evidence by not touching weapons, not moving any items unnecessarily, and by preventing unnecessary personnel from entering the crime scene. Your own personal safety is the ultimate priority. (3-1.2) (FR7 p. 50; FRASA pp. 24–25)

8.

C. Upon arriving at a crash scene, assess and observe the entire scene. Do not become focused on the vehicles or patients involved. Look to the right, left, above, and below the vehicle to ensure a safe scene. Remember that the area encompassing an accident scene can extend hundreds of feet in high-speed crashes. (3-1.2) (FR7 p. 50; FRASA p. 24)

9.

B. A patient who opens his eyes spontaneously is considered to be alert. To determine orientation, the patient must appropriately respond to inquiries into person, place, time, and self. You cannot determine if a patient is oriented by simple eye openings in response to verbal stimuli. Because this patient only opens his eyes when instructed to do so, he is considered to be responsive to verbal stimuli. (3-1.8) (FR7 p. 154; FRASA p. 216)

10.

B. All calls can be categorized as trauma or medical. If the First Responder rules out injury or the potential that an injury may have occurred, the call can typically be classified as a medical emergency. (3-1.4) (FR7 p. 138; FRASA p. 182)

11.

B. Falls, motor vehicle crashes, and shootings all involve injury or the potential for physical injury due to the mechanism of injury. A myocardial infarction is a true medical emergency that does not involve physical injury from a blunt or penetrating force. (3-1.4) (FR7 p. 147; FRASA p. 182)

12.

A. When you arrive at a scene and you determine there are more patients than one EMS unit can effectively manage, immediately call for additional assistance before making patient contact. If you make patient contact prior to calling for additional assistance, you may become focused on that one patient and not the whole scene. (3-1.6) (FR7 p. 148; FRASA p. 179)

13.

D. Determining the total number of patients is a major component of the scene size-up. Try to determine the total number of patients before making patient contact. The total number of patients will determine what additional resources are needed at the scene. (3-1.5) (FR7 p. 148; FRASA p. 179)

14.

D. Any requests for additional help and assistance should be made prior to patient contact if at all possible. If you wait until patient contact, you are likely to become focused on the patient's needs and not call for additional help. (3-1.6) (FR7 p. 148; p. 179)

15.

C. Categorization of the patient as being injured (trauma) is based primarily on the scene findings and the mechanism of injury. These two components of the scene size-up provide the preliminary information that allows you to categorize the patient into medical or trauma and determine priority of care. (3-1.4) (FR7 p. 141; FRASA pp. 182–183)

16.

A. Non-purposeful movement has no purpose relative to the painful (tactile) stimulation. A purposeful movement is one in which the patient makes an active attempt to remove the source of painful stimulation. There are two types of non-purposeful movement. Decorticate (flexion) posturing is when the patient arches the back and flexes the arms towards the chest. Decerebrate (extension) posturing is when the patient arches the back and extends the arms parallel to the body. (3-1.8) (FR7 p. 154; FRASA pp. 216–217)

17.

B. An alert adult who is gasping for air, is unable to speak, or has stridor indicates some type of partial airway obstruction. (3-1.10) (FR7 p. 169; FRASA p. 218)

18.

B. If you suspect the patient may have an injured spine, you must provide in-line spinal stabilization prior to continuing with the assessment. The patient may have fallen down the stairs. If you were to ask the patient questions before stabilizing the spine, the patient would likely look toward the person speaking to him or her, thus compromising the spine. (3-1.7) (FR7 pp. 142–143; FRASA p. 215, 217)

19.

D. The most effective way to determine if a patient is breathing is by looking at the patient's chest for chest rise and fall and listening and feeling for air exchange over the patient's mouth and nose. (3-1.10) (FR7 p. 156; FRASA p. 218)

20.

A. Your initial action for a patient who is not breathing is to provide immediate positive pressure ventilation. Delaying positive pressure ventilation will likely result in brain damage or cardiac arrest. (3-1.11) (FR7 p. 105, 156; FRASA p. 219)

21.

B. After ensuring an adequate airway, assess the patient's breathing status. If in doubt as to the adequacy of the breathing, provide positive pressure ventilation. Applying a gauze pad is not appropriate for an open chest wound. (3-1.10) (FR7 p. 105; FRASA p. 219)

22.

C. The patient may be presenting with a sign of a tension pneumothorax, a serious chest injury. You should release the occlusive dressing that is covering the sucking chest wound. (3-1.11) (FR7 pp. 335–336; FRASA p. 224, 353)

23.

D. The patient is potentially suffering from a head injury. The patient requires hyperventilation at 20 ventilations per minute if he is displaying signs of brain herniation such as a fixed and dilated pupil, non-purposeful posturing, and paralysis to one side. Cover the right ear loosely with a sterile dressing. (3-1.17) (FRASA p. 113)

24.

D. Your initial response to an obstructed airway from a foreign body in the infant is to deliver five rapid back slaps. These back slaps are delivered to the infant while supporting his or her body over your hand and knee. Chest thrusts are delivered after the back slaps. Never administer abdominal thrusts to an infant. Blind finger sweeps are not performed on the infant because this procedure may lodge the foreign body farther into the airway. (3-1.11) (FR7 p. 122; FRASA pp. 139–140)

25.

B. An infant is able to recognize his or her parent or primary caregiver at around 2 months. The infant will typically become agitated, may cry, and will look around to find the parent or caregiver. If the infant shows no response when removed from the parent or primary caregiver, it is an indication of a decreased mental status. (3-1.9) (FR7 p. 462; FRASA p. 497)

26.

B. In the adult patient you will first palpate the radial pulse, whereas in an infant the brachial artery in the upper arm is assessed. The carotid artery in the adult and femoral artery in the infant are assessed when the peripheral pulses are absent. (3-1.13) (FR7 p. 156–157; FRASA p. 219, 220)

27.

A. Blood flowing from a wound at a steady continuous flow is considered major bleeding. You should immediately apply direct pressure to the wound with a gloved hand. Most bleeding can be controlled by direct pressure. Once the bleeding is controlled, you should apply a pressure dressing. (3-1.14) (FR7 pp. 289; FRASA p. 330)

28.

D. You might expect a patient who has lost a significant amount of blood to present with cool skin. Cool skin is usually a sign of hypoperfusion (shock), a condition which can result from significant blood loss. Hot skin usually indicates hyperthermia (heat emergency). Cold skin is found in hypothermia (cold emergency). (3-1.12) (FR7 p. 159; FRASA p. 329)

29.

C. Capillary refill is most reliable in the infant or child less than 6 years of age. It can be quickly checked in the nail bed, the fleshy part of the palm along the ulnar margin, forehead, or cheeks. Capillary refill is usually less than 2 seconds. (3-1.12) (FR7 p. 157; FRASA pp. 203)

30.

A. The mechanism of injury may not be very apparent or well understood upon arrival at the scene. You should reconsider the mechanism of injury during the physical exam to reevaluate whether it was enough to cause critical injuries. (3-1.16) (FR7 p. 160; FRASA p. 183)

31.

B. Falls, if greater than 10 feet, bicycle collisions, and a motor vehicle collision where a person in the same passenger compartment as the patient has died are all considered significant. Low-speed motor vehicle collisions are not considered significant. (3-1.4) (FR7 p. 160)

32.
A. The patient with a significant mechanism of injury requires an initial assessment, followed by a head-to-toe physical exam, and then a SAMPLE history. (3-1.16) (FR7 p. 160; FRASA p. 214)

33.
A. The first step in the assessment of any patient following scene size-up is performing an initial assessment. The initial assessment is followed by the physical exam. The SAMPLE history followed by the ongoing assessment is the next step. (3-1.16) (FR7 p. 143; FRASA p. 198)

34.
D. The First Responder physical exam may be a focused exam of an area of a specific injury or it may be a head-to-toe exam looking for other injuries to the patient. The type of physical exam is dependent on the injury and patient condition. (3-1.16) (FR7 p. 158; FRASA p. 221)

35.
C. The type of assessment that is performed on a trauma patient is based on the mechanism of injury (MOI) and initial assessment findings. If the patient suffered a significant mechanism of injury, altered mental status, or possibility of multiple injuries, then a rapid head-to-toe assessment is performed. (3-1.16) (FR7 p. 158; FRASA pp. 221)

36.
D. Immediately perform a head-to-toe physical exam to determine if a life-threatening injury or condition exists. (3-1.16) (FR7 p. 171; FRASA pp. 221–222)

37.
D. An exam that is performed on the injured or ill patient to identify life-threatening injuries is called a First Responder head-to-toe physical exam. (3-1.16) (FR7 p. 159; FRASA pp. 221–222)

38.
C. A patient who has a significant mechanism of injury or an altered mental status requires a rapid head-to-toe physical exam. Because this patient is not oriented to place, he is considered to have an altered mental status. (3-1.15) (FR7 p. 160; FRASA pp. 221–222)

39.
C. DOTS is the mnemonic for deformities, open injuries, tenderness, and swelling. These are signs of injury that should be identified during your assessment. (3-1.17) (FRASA p. 223)

40.
C. The First Responder physical exam for an adult uses a systematic approach, starting at the head and proceeding down the neck, chest, abdomen, lower extremities, upper extremities, and finally the posterior body. (3-1.16) (FR7 pp. 171–176; FRASA p. 223)

41.
C. Palpate the entire head and face, noting any tenderness or deformities. The immobilization device should not be removed to perform the physical exam. Gently palpate the skull with your hands flattened over the skull. This will prevent you from inadvertently pushing your fingertips into a skull fracture. (3-1.17) (FR7 p. 173; FRASA p. 223)

42.
D. If you find inadequate breathing while performing a physical exam, you must immediately stop the assessment and provide positive pressure ventilation. Management of the airway and breathing takes precedence over continued assessment. (3-1.11) (FR7 pp. 173–176; FRASA p. 218)

43.
A. Paradoxical chest wall movement associated with a flail segment is a critical injury affecting the patient's breathing and must be managed immediately. An open humerus fracture, unless it is associated with major bleeding, is not considered a life-threatening injury. A tibia fracture is not a life threat. (3-1.15) (FR7 p. 174; FRASA p. 218)

44.
B. The rapid head-to-toe physical exam is performed to determine if additional life-threatening injuries or conditions are present. Subsequent care and treatment will be based on this examination. (3-1.16) (FR7 p. 171; FRASA p. 221)

45.
A. In a medical patient, there is no mechanism of injury that will tell you about your patient's injuries. Therefore, you must act like a detective and look for any and all clues about the chief complaint.

Further assessment of the chief complaint is considered the history of the present illness. (3-1.16) (FR7 p. 153; FRASA p. 227)

46.

D. The OPQRST mnemonic allows you to rapidly and systematically gather more information about the chief complaint. The mnemonic stands for onset, provocation/palliation, quality, radiation, severity, and time for duration. (3-1.18) (FRASA p. 252)

47.

B. The mnemonic OPQRST stands for onset, provocation, quality, radiation, severity, and finally the length of time the patient has had the symptom. (3-1.18) (FRASA p. 252)

48.

A. Provocation determines what makes the pain worse, whereas palliation determines what makes the pain better. This provides the EMT with the information to help gauge the severity of the illness. A patient who complains of severe chest pain while sitting in a chair should concern the EMT more than the patient whose chest pain after shoveling the driveway was relieved with rest. (3-1.18) (FRASA p. 252)

49.

B. Radiation of pain describes if the pain or symptom moves or radiates. (3-1.18) (FRASA p. 252)

50.

A. When assessing the quality of a patient's pain, you should ask open-ended questions, such as "What does the pain feel like?" Asking leading questions, such as "Is the pain sharp or dull?" may lead to an inaccurate description. Questions regarding what makes the pain worse pertain to provocation and not to quality. Asking questions about when and how the pain began pertains to onset. (3-1.18) (FR7 p. 164; FRASA p. 254)

51.

A. Gather the history first in the responsive medical patient. The history will provide valuable information and must be obtained before the patient becomes potentially unresponsive. The history is followed by the physical exam and then the ongoing assessment. (3-1.16) (FR7 p. 159; FRASA p. 221)

52.

C. In the unresponsive medical patient, you perform a rapid head-to-toe physical exam to determine the possible nature of the medical illness. This is followed by the patient history and then the ongoing assessment. (3-1.16) (FR7 p. 159; FRASA p. 221)

53.

C. A patient is considered to be comatose or in a coma when he or she does not respond to any type of painful stimuli. This is a high-priority patient. (3-1.15) (FR7 p. 154; FRASA pp. 216–217)

54.

B. Valuable information is commonly obtained when inspecting the area around the unresponsive medical patient. The condition of the patient's environment, presence of home oxygen supply, the patient's position in a hospital bed, and patient's medications are a few examples. (3-1.16) (FR7 p. 148; FRASA p. 218)

55.

B. Unequal pupils are usually an indication of stroke or possible head injury. Changes in pupil size and reactivity are commonly associated with drug overdose, oxygen starvation (hypoxia), or adverse environmental conditions. (3-1.16) (FR7 p. 172; FRASA p. 274, 419)

56.

D. When you have determined that your patient is unresponsive or has an altered mental status during the initial assessment, your next assessment step would be to perform a rapid head-to-toe physical exam. The rapid head-to-toe physical exam may help to determine the possible nature of the medical illness. The status of the airway, breathing, and circulation is assessed and managed during the initial assessment. (3-1.16) (FR7 p. 159; FRASA pp. 222–223)

57.

D. The unresponsive medical patient should be placed in the left lateral recumbent position, also known as the recovery or coma position. This position will help to protect the airway from vomitus, blood, and other secretions. Be prepared to suction the airway if secretions are present. The Trendelenburg (shock) position is thought to help increase blood perfusion to the brain and vital organs; however, the use of this position is controversial and may not be allowed by your local medical direction. The semi-Fowler's position requires the patient to sit in a semi-reclined position, which may permit secretions and vomitus to enter the airway and lungs. The prone position (face down) will not permit you access to the patient's face and airway. (3-1.16) (FR7 p. 78; FRASA p. 100)

58.

B. You will initially assess the responsive medical patient by evaluating the complaint and signs and symptoms. You should perform a rapid head-to-toe physical exam on patients you find unresponsive. You should perform a focused medical exam in the responsive patient after you obtain a SAMPLE history. (3-1.16) (FR7 p. 149; FRASA p. 227)

59.

B. The purpose of the ongoing assessment is to monitor the patient and his or her injuries. The ongoing assessment assesses the airway, breathing, and circulation interventions and vital signs. The ongoing assessment is not designed to initially identify life threats. These should have been identified in the rapid trauma assessment. (3-1.20) (FR7 p. 178; FRASA p. 229)

60.

A. All critically injured patients should be reassessed at least every 5 minutes so that indicators of a worsening situation or an improvement can be rapidly noted. (3-1.20) (FR7 p. 178; FRASA p. 229)

61.

C. The initial assessment does not include taking the time to assess the abdomen. This survey rapidly identifies if there are problems with the airway, breathing, and circulation. The abdomen is assessed during the First Responder physical exam after the initial assessment is completed. (3-1.16) (FR7 p. 153; FRASA p. 214)

62.

D. The information gathered from a repeated ongoing assessment should always be compared with previous findings. This will help you determine the current patient status, know whether or not the treatment you are providing is helping the patient, and quickly identify a deteriorating patient status. It provides trends in the patient's condition that need to be reported to the receiving hospital personnel. (3-1.20) (FR7 p. 178; FRASA p. 229)

63.

C. When reassessing the stable patient, you should repeat the vital signs and assessment findings at least every 15 minutes. By reassessing and obtaining the vital signs frequently, you will assess the effectiveness of your treatment and find other problems that were not found earlier. (3-1.20) (FR7 p. 178; FRASA p. 229)

64.

B. The mnemonic used to assess the mental status of a patient is AVPU. A-alert: Is the patient awake, is the patient able to talk and respond? V-verbal: Does the patient respond to verbal stimulus? P-painful: Does the patient respond to painful stimulus? U-unresponsive: The patient does not respond to pain. (3-1.20) (FR7 p. 154; FRASA p. 216)

65.

B. A decrease in the pulse rate and pulse quality may indicate a head injury or severe hypoxia. These signs should alert you to other injuries or a need to change your treatment, like providing positive pressure ventilation. A low blood sugar level (hypoglycemia) usually presents with an increased heart rate. A heat-related emergency usually presents with an increased heart rate that may be very strong. As the condition continues, the heart rate remains high and the quality becomes poor. An allergic reaction (anaphylactic shock) presents with an increased heart rate that can be of poor quality. (3-1.20) (FR7 p. 168; FRASA p. 419)

66.

A. An ongoing assessment is done to detect any changes in the patient's condition, to detect any missed injuries or conditions, and to adjust your treatment as needed. The ongoing assessment may reveal that your patient's condition has worsened and that you must change your treatment. As a First Responder, you do not make a diagnosis. (3-1.20) (FR7 p. 178; FRASA p. 229)

67.

D. By waiting at least 1 full second, you are allowing time for the repeater to "open" the channel, preventing the initial part of your transmission from being cut. (3-1.21) (FRASA p. 237)

68.

B. By saying "Over" you are informing the receiver that you are through with your transmission. By waiting for confirmation, you are assured that the other party got your message and has no further questions. (3-1.21)

69.

C. It is very helpful to keep a standard format when communicating with responding EMS units. Use the following sequence when communicating with responding EMS units: 1) the patient's age and sex, 2) the patient's chief complaint, 3) patient's mental status, 4) airway and breathing status, and 5) the circulation status of the patient. In addition, you should determine the estimated time of arrival of the EMS unit or resources that are responding. (3-1.21) (FR7 p. 178; FRASA p. 239)

70.

A. After medical direction has given you an order, you should repeat the order back to medical direction word for word. Repeating the order back will help ensure that the order was given and received correctly. This is referred to as the "echo" method. If the person giving you the order has not identified himself or herself, you should ask for his or her name and document it on the run report. (3-1.21) (FRASA p. 239)

71.

A. The oral hand-off report should summarize the information you are reporting to the EMS crew when handing off patient care. It should include the following information and be done in the following sequence: 1) age and sex, 2) chief complaint, 3) responsiveness, 4) airway and breathing status, 5) circulation status, 6) physical exam findings, 7) SAMPLE history, and 8) interventions provided. (3-1.21) (FR7 p. 178; FRASA p. 230)

72.

B. By positioning yourself at the same level of the patient or lower, you help decrease the fear and anxiety of the patient. (3-1.9) (FR7 p. 456; FRASA p. 239)

73.

D. Elderly patients often have a higher threshold for pain and do not complain of pain until it is severe. Take any complaint of pain in an elderly patient very seriously. (*) (FRASA p. 527)

74.

C. Push the press-to-talk button and wait 1 second before transmitting. Speak with your mouth 2 to 3 inches from the microphone. After receiving orders from medical control, echo back the orders. Avoid making a diagnosis, and provide only objective information or important relevant, subjective information. (*) (FR7 p. 178; FRASA p. 237)

75.

A. If medical direction has given you an order that you feel is inappropriate, you should immediately question the order. It is possible that medical direction misunderstood something you said, or medical direction may have misspoken when giving the order. It is best to question the order in a professional manner. (*) (FRASA p. 239)

76.

D. While gathering your general impression of the injured patient, any life threats must be managed before proceeding with the assessment. An open wound to the chest must be immediately managed by placing your gloved hand directly over the wound site. (3-1.7) (FR7 p. 289; FRASA p. 330)

77.

D. Gunshot entrance wounds may be away from the spine; however, after the projectile enters the body, it can strike the spine. While forming your general impression of this patient before continuing your assessment, you must provide in-line stabilization of the spine. (3-1.7) (FR7 p. 146, 154; FRASA p. 215)

78.

B. When the mechanism of injury is significant, as it is with this patient, you should perform a rapid head-to-toe physical exam of the patient. The rapid trauma exam will help to identify other injuries such as additional gunshot wounds or exit wounds. The focused physical exam is completed when you do not suspect a significant mechanism of injury. The focused physical exam is the exam of the specific injury site. (3-1.16) (FR7 p. 159; FRASA p. 221)

79.

D. This is a rather minor example of maintaining patient confidentiality. Confidentiality is the patient's legal right, and it is your ethical responsibility not to divulge such information. (*) (FR7 p. 28; FRASA p. 41)

80.

B. The next immediate step in the assessment process is to determine if he responds to verbal stimuli. All you have determined at this point is that he is not alert. He may respond to your voice or command with appropriate communication that would provide information about his airway and breathing status. If he talks to you, there is no need to open the airway manually or to insert an airway adjunct. If he does not respond to verbal stimuli, you would then assess his response to painful stimuli. The pulse and skin check occurs after assessment of the breathing status. (3-1.8) (FR7 p. 154; FRASA p. 216)

81.

B. During the general impression of the initial assessment, you inspect for obvious life-threatening injuries that need immediate management. On approaching the patient, if you note a major bleed, such as spurting or steadily flowing blood, you or a partner should quickly expose the area and apply direct pressure. Once direct pressure is applied, you should then move on to the remainder of the initial assessment. Positive pressure ventilation is necessary in this patient; however, it will be performed after establishing the airway. Manual spinal stabilization is necessary and should be performed prior to establishing an airway. Oxygen administration is necessary; however, it will be delivered by positive pressure ventilation. A nonrebreather mask is not appropriate in this patient because it will not provide ventilation. (3-1.7) (FR7 p. 289; FRASA p. 330)

82.

A. There are several life threats that must be managed in this patient: the open wound to the chest, the blood in the mouth, the hypoxia, and the poor ventilation status. You must clear the airway immediately—prior to positive pressure ventilation—to prevent aspiration. A nonrebreather mask is not applied until after assessment of the ventilation status and only if the breathing status is determined to be adequate. In this patient, the ventilatory status is inadequate; therefore, oxygen should be delivered via the ventilation device. The gunshot wound to the chest must be occluded as quickly as possible. (3-1.11) (FR7 pp. 335–336; FRASA p. 218)

83.

A. All of the possible choices are signs or symptoms of a possible fracture. However, the most objective is crepitation. Crepitation is a grating sensation found when bone ends rub over each other. Pain, ecchymosis (discoloration), and edema (swelling) could all be found in ligament, tendon, or muscle injuries where there is no actual bone injury. (3-1.17) (FR7 p. 363; FRASA p. 461)

84.

A. Capillary refill does not provide as accurate information in the adult patient as in the infant and young child. The adult patient may have pre-existing -

disease conditions that may cause a delay. Research has found that some people have a normally slow capillary refill, some up to 4 seconds. Also, environmental conditions play a role in capillary refill. A cold environment, for example, will cause the refill to be delayed. (3-1.12) (FR7 p. 157; FRASA p. 203)

85.

C. During the general impression when you are attempting to ascertain the chief complaint, note the patient's speech pattern. A patient who says a few words and then must gasp for a breath is showing objective signs of respiratory distress. It would be normal for a patient who is crying loudly to gasp for a breath. Typically, patients who are having trouble breathing (dyspneic) sit upright or may be propped up in bed with a few pillows. Even though the patient is on 2 lpm of oxygen at home, that does not mean that he or she is dyspneic. (3-1.7) (FR7 pp. 168–169; FRASA p. 197)

86.

B. Because the respirations are shallow, indicating an inadequate tidal volume of air being breathed in, the priority of management of this patient is to establish an airway by employing a jaw-thrust maneuver followed by positive pressure ventilation. Application of a nonrebreather mask will not correct the inadequate tidal volume and will not correct the inadequate breathing status. A blood pressure will not be taken until after the airway and ventilation are managed and the initial assessment and rapid trauma assessment are completed. It is more important to establish an airway prior to ventilation than to apply a dressing to a moderately bleeding wound. Only severe bleeding is managed during the initial assessment. (3-1.11) (FR7 p. 102; FRASA p. 99)

87.

D. Because the patient has the potential for multiple injuries based on the mechanism of injury, a rapid head-to-toe physical exam must be conducted. A focused physical exam is used only if there is no possible chance of other injuries. A detailed exam may be conducted by the EMS crew after they have conducted a rapid trauma assessment. The patient should not be allowed to drive to the hospital based on her injuries. (3-1.16) (FR7 p. 159; FRASA p. 221)

88.

B. All of the choices must be performed on this patient; however, the first priority is to ensure your own safety. Do not get drawn into dramatic scenes without first conducting a scene size-up to be sure safety hazards have been identified and managed. (3-1.1) (FRASA p. 179)

89.

C. The airway has been secured; therefore, the next immediate action is to begin positive pressure ventilation. Even though the rate is adequate, the tidal volume is not. An inadequate rate or tidal volume is an indication of inadequate breathing. Inadequate breathing is treated by providing positive pressure ventilation. Application of a nonrebreather mask will provide an increased amount of oxygen to the patient; however, most of the oxygen will not reach the alveoli because the volume is inadequate. Chest compressions are not indicated because the patient still has pulses. A cervical spinal immobilization collar will be applied during the head-to-toe physical exam, not during the initial assessment. (3-1.10) (FR7 pp. 104–105; FRASA pp. 103, 106)

90.

A. The patient is complaining orally when you arrive on the scene; therefore, you should assume the airway is open and the breathing is adequate. These are both parts of the initial assessment. To complete the initial assessment, you must assess the circulation by checking the pulses and skin color, temperature, and condition. (1-3.12) (FR7 p. 153; FRASA p. 214)

91.

B. Because the patient is a minor, consent becomes an issue of concern. However, because the patient has suffered a critical injury, it is necessary to initiate emergency care under implied consent. In the case of a minor injury, it would be prudent to attempt to contact the parents or legal guardian of the child prior to transport. (3-1.15) (FR7 p. 23; FRASA p. 36)

92.

A. During the general impression of the initial assessment, it is necessary to manage any obvious major bleeding. Because the bleeding has been identified by the patient, you should quickly assess the foot and determine if the bleeding is spurting or flowing steadily from the wound. If so, this would be considered a major bleed and you must then control the bleeding. If not, you would proceed with the initial assessment and assess the circulation because the airway is patent and breathing is adequate, as evidenced by the patient's oral complaints and speech pattern. (3-1.15) (FR7 pp. 156–157; FRASA p. 328)

93.

D. Following the initial assessment, you should next perform a rapid head-to-toe physical exam because the patient has an altered mental status. If the patient were coherent, it would be appropriate to conduct a focused physical exam and SAMPLE history. (3-1.16) (FR7 p. 159; FRASA p. 221)

94.

C. You would approach the patient from the front of the vehicle if possible and instruct the patient not to move his head or neck. You or your partner would then gain access to the vehicle and provide manual stabilization of the spine while in the vehicle. Once that is done, you would then proceed with the general impression and the remainder of the initial assessment. (3-1.4) (FR7 p. 142; FRASA p. 215)

95.

C. The patient obviously has an altered mental status; therefore, he could be deemed unable to make a rational decision. Based on implied consent, you would assess the patient and begin emergency care. (3-1.8) (FR7 p. 23; FRASA p. 36)

96.

D. Capillary refill is most accurate in younger children. It is used to assess the perfusion status of the patient. Capillary refill is subject to environmental influences such as cold weather that would cause the vessels in the periphery to constrict, thereby reducing the blood flow to that area. This would cause the capillary refill to be reduced. The asthma patient is suffering a ventilation problem, not a perfusion problem. It is appropriate to assess capillary refill in the 30-year-old who was shot in the chest; however, it has been found that the capillary refill test is most accurate in younger children. (3-1.12) (FR7 p. 157; FRASA p. 203)

97.

A. Blood mixed with clear fluid coming from the ears, nose, or mouth is likely blood mixed with cerebrospinal fluid. This is typically an indication of a skull fracture. A "halo test" can be performed to determine if the blood is mixed with cerebrospinal fluid. This is where blood is dropped onto a cotton gauze pad or pillow case. The cerebrospinal fluid forms a yellow ring around the blood in the center of the cotton cloth. This test has limited usefulness since research has found that saliva and saline will also cause the same result. (3-1.17) (FR7 p. 173; FRASA p. 422)

98.

D. The gurgling sound indicates that the patient has blood, vomitus, secretions, or some other substance in the airway. This requires immediate suction. Also, the patient has a respiratory rate of only 6/minute, which indicates inadequate breathing. After clearing the airway, positive pressure ventilation must be initiated. (3-1.11) (FR7 p. 129; FRASA p. 101)

99.

C. The respiratory rate of a newborn may be 40–60/minute. As the infant grows older, the respiratory rate declines. Once the child reaches adolescence, the respiratory rate is close to that of an adult. (3-1.11) (FR7 p. 157; FRASA p. 96)

100.

C. Because the patient is responsive, the next step is to gather a SAMPLE history and then perform a focused physical exam in which you would examine the abdomen and other related body systems. You would have already determined the level of responsiveness during the initial assessment. Also, it appears the patient is continuing to complain, indicating the mental status has not changed. A rapid head-to-toe exam would be performed if the patient were unresponsive or had an altered mental status. (3-1.16) (FR7 p. 159; FRASA p. 227)

101.

C. The skin is the best indicator of the patient's perfusion status. During the initial assessment you are trying to identify a life threat to the circulation. (3-1.12) (FR7 p. 159; FRASA p. 334)

102.

A. All of the injuries, except for the fractured ribs, would be considered possible life threats. If two or more ribs were fractured in two or more places creating a flail segment, it would be considered a life-threatening injury. However, simple rib fractures are not life threatening unless they lacerate the lung or another underlying organ. Femur fractures and pelvis fractures have a tendency to bleed severely from the fractured bone itself. An open wound to the posterior thorax can lead to a significant amount of air trapped in the pleural space, causing the lung to collapse. This would lead to a compromise in gas exchange and hypoxia. (3-1.15) (FR7 p. 174; FRASA pp. 373, 465–471)

103.

A. The patient's airway is open, the breathing is adequate, and his pulse is present. Since he has an altered mental status, you would apply a nonrebreather mask if available and perform a rapid head-to-toe physical exam. There is no need for spinal stabilization since there is no mechanism of trauma that would indicate a possible spine injury. The breathing is adequate; therefore, there is no need for artificial ventilation. (3-1.16) (FR7 p. 159; FRASA p. 221)

104.

C. The skin is warm and dry and normal in color. This would indicate good tissue perfusion. Hypovolemic shock would result in poor tissue perfusion in which the skin would be pale, cool, and clammy. Hypoxia and inadequate delivery of hemoglobin would cause cyanosis. (3-1.12) (FR7 p. 159; FRASA pp. 219–220)

105.

C. The unresponsive medical patient should be placed in a left lateral recumbent position. This is also known as the coma or recovery position. This position is used to allow secretions and vomit to drain from the mouth and airway. (3-1.11) (FR7 p. 78; FRASA p. 100)

106.

D. Pain is a subjective complaint. You cannot assess and objectively determine if the pain really exists or not. A symptom is a complaint of the patient. The others are all signs. You can observe or palpate a deformed extremity, heart rate, or excessive neck muscle use. (*) (FR7 p. 159; FRASA p. 227)

107.

D. The first priority is to determine if the scene is safe. The best person at a building collapse to determine the safety hazard of further collapse is the engineer. (1-3.3) (FR7 p. 502; FRASA p. 179)

108.

C. Once the scene is cleared of safety hazards, you would approach the patient, apply manual spinal stabilization, quickly assess the posterior thorax, and logroll the patient into a supine position. (1-3.7) (FR7 p. 81; FRASA pp. 444, 447)

109.

C. A patient who is found in a fetal position is most likely suffering from severe abdominal pain. The fetal position relieves some of the tension of the abdominal wall muscles and places less pressure on the underlying organs. Appendicitis may produce severe abdominal pain. (1-3.7) (FR7 p. 252; FRASA p. 277))

110.
C. Because the patient has an altered mental status, you must treat him under implied consent. It would be best to have law enforcement present to assist and witness the restraint process. Do not restrain the patient in a prone position. This may interfere with his airway and impede his ventilation. (1-3.3) (FR7 p. 23; FRASA p. 36)

111.
D. A car on its roof is considered an unstable vehicle. It is possible that the car may collapse under the weight, thus making it unsafe. The fire department must stabilize the vehicle prior to your entry. (3-1.3) (FR7 p. 509; FRASA pp. 587–588)

112.
A. An unresponsive patient with a fixed and dilated pupil following trauma to his head is most likely suffering from a brain injury with compression and herniation of brain tissue. A patient who is responsive and who has a fixed and dilated pupil is not suffering from herniation of the brain. He is more likely suffering from an injury to the eye itself or an injury to the third cranial nerve. (1-3.17) (FR7 p. 172; FRASA p. 204)

113.
A. A rigid and tender abdomen is a sign of bleeding within the abdominal cavity (intra-abdominal bleeding). Pale, cool, clammy skin and weak rapid radial pulses are indications of poor perfusion. (1-3.17) (FR7 p. 174; FRASA p. 277)

114.
B. The abdominal cavity is covered by a peritoneal lining. Blood leaking into the peritoneal cavity will cause irritation of the lining. The irritation will cause abdominal pain, tenderness on palpation, and abdominal wall guarding and rigidity. (3-1.17) (FR7 p. 174; FRASA p. 377)

115.
B. Palliation refers to any relief or alleviation of the symptom. Palliation of the breathing difficulty in this patient is achieved by an upright position. (3-1.19) (FRASA p. 252)

116.
C. Tenderness and pain on palpation of the symphysis pubis usually indicates a pelvic fracture. When assessing the pelvis, if the patient is already complaining of pain prior to palpation, do not palpate. If not, press down and then inward on the anterior iliac crest, assessing for a pain response, instability, and crepitus. You should then apply pressure to the symphysis pubis. (3-1.17) (FR7 p. 175, 358; FRASA p. 225)

117.
C. A patient with abdominal discomfort and pelvic pain may be suffering from a pelvic fracture and intra-abdominal bleeding. This patient is considered unstable; therefore, you should conduct an ongoing assessment every 5 minutes. (3-1.20) (FR7 p. 178; FRASA p. 229)

118.
C. Assessment of the ears and nose in the chest pain patient would be the least relevant to check. The oral mucosa may provide information about the oxygenation status. Inspection of the chest is important to assess for potential evidence of injury to the chest causing the complaint of chest pain. The pedal pulses will provide information about the perfusion status. (*) (FR7 pp. 173–176; FRASA pp. 223–226)

119.
B. To ensure that you have properly transferred the care of the patient to the emergency department, you must provide an oral report to medical personnel who are of equal or higher level of training than yourself. Until that official transfer of care is done, you must remain with the patient, even in the emergency department. (*) (FR7 p. 27; FRASA p. 39)

120.
D. A fall of less than two times the height of the patient is not considered to be a significant mechanism of trauma. A fall of greater than two times the height of the patient would be considered a significant mechanism of injury. (3-1.4) (FR7 p. 160; FRASA pp. 182–183)

121.
C. A component of the scene size-up is to determine the number of patients and call for additional resources. If several patients are found upon entering the scene, you should call for additional resources at that time. (1-3.5) (FR7 p. 526; FRASA p. 559)

122.

B. Because the laceration of the leg could be a wound with major bleeding, it is necessary to immediately expose the extremity and inspect the wound. Obvious life threats such as major bleeding, vomitus in the airway, and open wounds to the chest are managed as part of the general impression. Once the bleeding is controlled, you would continue with the initial assessment. (1-3.14) (FR7 p. 319; FRASA p. 330)

123.

C. Dizziness and weakness in a diabetic patient are not indications of an immediate life threat or a priority status. In many diabetic patients, the dizziness and weakness may be related to an episode of hypoglycemia. Administration of glucose will reverse the symptoms. The other selections are all priority indicators. (1-3.15) (FR7 pp. 247–248; FRASA pp. 269–270)

124.

B. Discoloration to the mastoid process is also known as Battle's sign. It typically indicates a posterior basilar skull fracture. The discoloration, however, does not occur usually for several hours after the injury. (1-3.17) (FR7 p. 397; FRASA p. 422)

125.

B. It is difficult to assess a blood pressure in children less than 3 years of age. It is more important to rely on peripheral and central pulses and the skin signs to determine perfusion status. It would be difficult to assess the orientation in a 2-year-old patient. The reddened sclera does not apply to a dehydrated patient. (1-3.13) (FR7 p. 480; FRASA pp. 504–506)

126.

B. A patient with an altered mental status may not be able to control his or her own airway. Therefore, it is important that in any patient with an altered mental status you carefully assess and monitor the airway. (1-3.8) (FR7 p. 154; FRASA p. 216)

127.

C. Scene safety is your first concern. Until the scene is determined to be safe, you should remain in the first-response vehicle. (1-3.2) (FR7 p. 48; FRASA pp. 181–182)

128.

B. During exhalation, the chest wall is moving inward. A segment that moves opposite or outward when the remainder of the chest is moving inward would be considered to be moving in a paradoxical motion. This is an indication of a flail segment. (1-3.17) (FR7 p. 100; FRASA p. 218)

129.

D. Stridor is a high-pitched sound that is produced from air rushing past a partial obstruction at the level of the larynx. It is commonly produced by swelling that occurs in the larynx. (1-3.10) (FR7 p. 113; FRASA p. 135)

130.

D. Because the patient is talking when you arrive at her side, you have already determined she is alert, her airway is patent, and her breathing is adequate. The next step in the initial assessment is to assess the pulse and skin. (1-3.12) (FR7 p. 153; FRASA p. 219)

131.

B. A patient with hot, dry skin may be suffering from a heat-related emergency such as heat stroke. This is a dire emergency that requires rapid treatment and transport. Shock and heart attack normally produce cool and diaphoretic skin. A stroke usually presents with no significant skin findings. (1-3.17) (FR7 pp. 262–263; FRASA p. 294–296)

132.

D. Any female patient in child-bearing years who is complaining of abdominal pain should be questioned about her menstrual period. You want to determine if she has missed a period, if any abnormal discharge has occurred, bleeding between the periods, or if the period was excessively heavy. This may provide you with a clue that the condition may be related to a reproductive organ injury or disorder. (1-3.19) (FR7 p. 252; FRASA p. 276, 486)

133.

C. The patient has tachycardia. A heart rate greater than 100 bpm in an adult patient is considered to be tachycardia. A narrow pulse pressure is when the difference between the systolic and diastolic blood pressure is less than 30 mmHg. Tachypnea is a respiratory rate that is greater than 20 per minute in the adult. Hypertension is defined as a systolic blood pressure greater than 160 mmHg and a diastolic greater than 90 mmHg. (*) (FR7 p. 168)

134.

D. Apply an occlusive dressing to any wound to the thorax. Regardless if the wound is anterior (front), lateral (side), or posterior (back), it may still be a sucking chest wound. This type of wound could easily produce a tension pneumothorax (collapsed lung due to extreme pressure built up in the chest). (1-3.17) (FR7 p. 297; FRASA p. 353)

135.

B. The medical term for swelling is edema. Erythema is redness. Ecchymosis means discoloration of a black and blue tint. A contusion is a bruise. (*) (FR7 p. 587; FRASA pp. 244, 588)

136.

A. Because aspiration would interfere with gas exchange in the alveoli and produce hypoxia, pale, cool, clammy skin would be an early sign. Cyanosis would be a later sign of severe hypoxia. (1-3.10) (FRASA p. 202)

137.

D. Even if the patient refuses, attempt to persuade the patient to allow you to assess her. It is important to be sure that you inform the patient of the possible consequences of the possible injuries. (*) (FR7 p. 21; FRASA p. 37)

138.

C. A systemic allergic reaction, also known as anaphylaxis, will cause the bronchioles to constrict and become inflamed on the internal surface. This increase in airway resistance will produce wheezing when air rushes through. Another hallmark sign is hives, and a symptom is itching. (*) (FR7 p. 261; FRASA pp. 338–339)

139.

D. Approximately 50 percent of the patients who suffer a tonic-clonic (generalized) seizure will bite their tongue. If you arrive on the scene of a patient who has suffered an altered mental status and a laceration to the tongue, you should suspect a possible seizure. (1-3.17) (FR7 p. 246; FRASA 276)

140.

B. All patients, regardless of how serious or minor the extent of the injury or illness, must have an initial assessment. (1-3.7) (FR7 p. 138; FRASA p. 198)

141.

A. The purpose of the rapid head-to-toe physical exam is to identify and manage life threats to the patient. (1-3.16) (FR7 p. 159; FRASA p. 220)

142.

C. When a patient says a few words and then must gasp for a breath, it is a good indication that the patient is having difficulty breathing. A crying patient, or one who talks with a completely normal speech pattern, typically is not having a difficult time breathing. (1-3.10) (FR7 p. 239; FRASA pp. 101–103)

143.

B. A fall from the roof of a house would be an indication to suspect a spinal injury. Therefore, it is necessary to take manual spinal stabilization prior to proceeding in the initial assessment. (1-3.4) (FR7 p. 101; FRASA p. 215)

144.

D. The patient has inadequate respirations. Because the patient is not responding to painful stimuli, you can insert an oropharyngeal airway to facilitate maintaining an open airway and begin ventilation with a pocket mask or BVM. (1-3.11) (FR7 p. 126; FRASA p. 103)

145.

B. Tenderness is pain on palpation. Rigidity is an involuntary abdominal muscle contraction. Guarding is voluntary abdominal muscle contraction. Pain is a patient complaint that occurs without any palpation or manipulation of the area. (1-3.1) (FR7 p. 174; FRASA pp. 276–277)

4 Circulation Emergencies

module objectives

Questions in this module relate to D.O.T.
objectives 4-1.1 to 4-1.11

DIRECTIONS

Each of the questions or incomplete statements below is followed by suggested answers or completions. Select the **one answer** that is best in each case.

1. Which of the following would most likely cause the heart to stop beating?
   A. fractures
   B. low blood sugar level
   C. blocked coronary artery
   D. fever

2. The most common cause of cardiac arrest in infants and young children is:
   A. heart attack.
   B. stroke.
   C. congenital heart defect.
   D. airway or breathing disturbance.

3. Which of the following is **not** a component of basic cardiopulmonary resuscitation?
   A. administration of medications
   B. compression of the chest
   C. positive pressure ventilation
   D. establishing responsiveness

4. A bystander witnesses an adult patient fall to the ground and become unresponsive. He should first perform which step?
   A. Call 911.
   B. Perform one-person CPR.
   C. Seek a defibrillator.
   D. Try to identify an advanced-level provider.

5. Blood is ejected from the right atrium to the:
   A. right ventricle to the lungs to the aorta.
   B. left ventricle to the lungs to the left atrium.
   C. right ventricle to the lungs to the left atrium to the left ventricle.
   D. left ventricle to the lungs to the right ventricle to the left atrium.

6. The site where the exchange of oxygen, carbon dioxide, and other vital nutrients takes place is in the:
   A. large arteries.
   B. capillaries.
   C. arterioles.
   D. venules.

7. The heart can be divided into two separate pumps:
   A. the low-pressure left myocardium and the high-pressure right myocardium.
   B. the high-pressure right myocardium and the high-pressure left myocardium.
   C. the low-pressure right myocardium and the high-pressure left myocardium.
   D. the low-pressure right myocardium and the low-pressure left myocardium.

SCENARIO

Questions 8–12 refer to the following scenario:

You are called to the scene for a possible cardiac arrest. Dispatch informs you that the wife of the patient heard him fall and immediately called 911. The male patient is 56 years of age. You arrive on the scene and find a male patient lying on the kitchen floor. He is not moving and appears to be cyanotic.

8. Your first immediate action is to:
   A. open the airway.
   B. assess for breathing.
   C. establish unresponsiveness.
   D. check for a carotid pulse.

9. After you have performed the above, the next immediate action you should perform is to:
   A. open the airway.
   B. assess for breathing.
   C. establish unresponsiveness.
   D. check for a carotid pulse.

10. What pulse would you check on this patient?
    A. radial
    B. carotid
    C. pedal
    D. brachial

11. You determine that the patient is not breathing and the pulse is absent. You should immediately begin chest compressions and ventilation at a ratio of _____ compressions to _____ ventilation(s).
    A. 5, 1
    B. 30, 2
    C. 15, 1
    D. 15, 2

12. While performing one-person CPR on the patient, you should deliver _____ compressions in 1 minute.
    A. 60
    B. 80
    C. 100
    D. 120

13. When delivering ventilation to the patient in cardiac arrest, if no oxygen is connected to the ventilation device, a tidal volume of _____ should be delivered with each ventilation.
    A. 3–4 ml/kg
    B. 6–7 ml/kg
    C. 10 ml/kg
    D. 20 ml/kg

14. When performing chest compression on an adult patient, the sternum should be compressed approximately:
    A. $\frac{1}{2}$–1 inch.
    B. $1\frac{1}{2}$–2 inches.
    C. 2–$2\frac{1}{2}$ inches.
    D. one-third the depth of the chest.

15. The proper landmark for finger position for chest compression on the infant is:
    A. heel of the hand on lower half of the sternum.
    B. heel of both hands on lower half of the sternum.
    C. two fingers one finger's width below the intermammary line.
    D. two fingers one finger's width above the intermammary line.

16. Which of the following best describes proper compressions for a 5-year-old patient in cardiac arrest?
    A. heel of one hand on the lower half of the sternum compressing $1\frac{1}{2}$–2 inches
    B. heel of both hands on lower half of the sternum compressing one-third to one-half the depth of the chest
    C. two fingers placed one finger's width below the intermammary line compressing one-third to one-half the depth of the chest
    D. heel of one or two hands on the lower half of the sternum compressing one-third to one-half the depth of the sternum

17. The compression-to-ventilation ratio for a 3-year-old in cardiac arrest is _____ compressions to _____ ventilation(s).
    A. 15, 2
    B. 15, 1
    C. 30, 2
    D. 5, 2

18. While you are performing one-person CPR, a second First Responder arrives on the scene. The second rescuer should:
    A. immediately begin ventilation.
    B. assess for effectiveness of compressions by feeling for a carotid pulse.
    C. have you stop compressions immediately and begin the count where you left off.
    D. begin to ventilate the patient after every fifth compression.

19. When delivering a ventilation to a 7-year-old, the ventilation should be delivered over:
    A. 4 seconds.
    B. 2 seconds.
    C. 1 second.
    D. $\frac{1}{2}$ second.

20. Which of the following would be an acceptable indication for the First Responder to stop cardiopulmonary resuscitation?
    A. when he or she feels the patient is no longer viable
    B. when the pulse can no longer be felt with compressions
    C. when the patient is delivered to the EMS crew
    D. when the patient's color remains cyanotic

AUTOMATED EXTERNAL DEFIBRILLATION AND EMERGENCY CARDIAC CARE

21. The automated external defibrillator (AED) should be applied to which patient?
    A. a 6-year-old patient in cardiac arrest
    B. a 17-year-old patient in traumatic cardiac arrest
    C. a 55-year-old patient whose chief complaint is chest pain
    D. a 43-year-old patient who is unresponsive, pulseless, and apneic

22. Your patient complains of shortness of breath and has a history of congestive heart failure. What is the most likely position of comfort the patient will want to be placed in?
    A. supine position
    B. Trendelenberg position
    C. sitting up
    D. left lateral recumbent position

23. Within the first 8 minutes, what is the most common presenting rhythm in cardiac arrest?
    A. asystole
    B. ventricular tachycardia
    C. ventricular fibrillation
    D. pulseless electrical activity

24. The most effective treatment for ventricular fibrillation in an unwitnessed arrest is:
    A. immediate defibrillation.
    B. hyperventilation.
    C. CPR and then defibrillation.
    D. rapid transport.

25. If you are the only First Responder on the scene and have an AED, prior to leaving the patient to call for additional help, you should deliver:
    A. two sets of three shocks totaling six.
    B. as many shocks as needed to convert the patient out of ventricular fibrillation.
    C. one shock.
    D. one set of three shocks.

26. After the AED is used, a case review would be beneficial for all the following reasons **except:**
    A. improving CPR and determining if steps can be taken to decrease the time to defibrillation.
    B. determining how to work more effectively with ALS crews.
    C. determining if the AED is effective in converting ventricular fibrillation to a perfusing rhythm.
    D. determining if further training is needed and in what areas.

27. Once you reach the side of a patient who is pulseless and apneic, the first shock in a witnessed arrest from the AED should be delivered in less than:
    A. 1 minute.
    B. 2 minutes.
    C. 3 minutes.
    D. 4 minutes.

28. The most common cause of failure of the AED is due to:
    A. electronic malfunction.
    B. improper placement of the pads.
    C. patient artifact.
    D. a dead battery.

29. By completing the operator checklist, you are assured of all of the following **except:**
    A. the batteries are fully charged.
    B. the cables are in working condition.
    C. the operator is proficient in the use of the AED.
    D. appropriate defibrillation pads are available.

30. To be most effective in converting ventricular fibrillation into a perfusing rhythm, defibrillation should occur within _____ of the cardiac arrest?
    A. 10 minutes
    B. 8 minutes
    C. 6 minutes
    D. 4 minutes

31. If proper CPR is being performed, defibrillation may be successful for up to _____ after the onset of cardiac arrest.
    A. 10 minutes
    B. 8 minutes
    C. 6 minutes
    D. 12 minutes

32. After delivering a defibrillation, a pulse check should be performed:
    A. immediately after the defibrillation.
    B. after delivering 2 ventilations.
    C. only prior to the next defibrillation.
    D. after 5 cycles of CPR.

33. How can you effectively allow for the chest to completely recoil after each chest compression?:
    A. Remove your hands from the patient's chest after each compression.
    B. Maintain steady downward pressure on the chest.
    C. Bring your hands completely up after each compression.
    D. Ventilate with greater force and higher volume.

34. Circumstances that may lead to inappropriate defibrillation include all of the following **except:**
    A. placing the AED on a patient who is complaining of chest pain.
    B. placing the AED on a patient in ventricular tachycardia who has a pulse.
    C. placing the AED on a patient who is pulseless and apneic.
    D. mechanical failure caused by poorly maintained or faulty batteries.

35. After successfully defibrillating your patient, you are waiting for the EMS crew. You have applied oxygen and left the AED on the patient. Your patient suddenly becomes pulseless and apneic. You should immediately:
    A. begin chest compressions.
    B. press the analyze button to analyze the patient rhythm.
    C. insert an oropharyngeal airway and begin ventilation.
    D. remove the AED pads and do not deliver any additional shocks.

36. A patient who was previously defibrillated and regained a pulse loses his pulse and deteriorates into ventricular fibrillation. You should:
    A. begin CPR and call for EMS transport.
    B. shock the patient once.
    C. deliver three stacked shocks.
    D. do nothing and the ventricular fibrillation will likely convert on its own.

37. How often should you reassess the patient following a successful resuscitation?
    A. when the patient begins to experience chest pain
    B. only once before the EMS crew arrives
    C. at least every 5 minutes or whenever the patient's condition changes
    D. every 15 minutes if the patient's condition does not change

38. Any time the semiautomatic defibrillator advises "No Shock" and the patient is pulseless, you should:

    A. stop and turn the machine off.

    B. disconnect the leads from the AED, leaving only the patches in place on the patient's chest.

    C. perform CPR for 2 minutes and then check the pulse and re-analyze the rhythm.

    D. turn the machine off and then back on to reset the analyzing unit.

39. Which of the following is a contraindication for application and use of an AED?

    A. an 80-year-old cardiac arrest patient

    B. a child less than 1 year of age

    C. a patient with a recent history of open-heart surgery

    D. a patient between 1 and 8 years of age

40. You arrive on the scene and find a 66-year-old female patient complaining of chest discomfort only that is a 4 on a scale of 1 to 10. Her respirations are 18 per minute and her chest is rising adequately with each breath. Which of the following would be the most appropriate oxygen therapy device and liter flow for this patient?

    A. nasal cannula at 2 lpm

    B. nonrebreather mask at 15 lpm

    C. nasal cannula at 10 lpm

    D. nonrebreather mask at 6 lpm

41. You are preparing to assess a 68-year-old patient who was complaining of chest tightness. You should assess the patient in which order?

    A. breathing, circulation, skin, airway, mental status

    B. general impression, airway, circulation, mental status, skin, breathing

    C. breathing, airway, circulation, skin

    D. general impression, mental status, airway, breathing, circulation, skin

42. What term is used for a patient who suffers a heart attack in which he or she never experiences the typical chest pain or discomfort?

    A. silent heart attack

    B. muted heart attack

    C. tranquil heart attack

    D. quiet heart attack

43. You arrive on the scene and find a 42-year-old responsive patient who is experiencing cardiac compromise. Your first assessment concern is:

    A. pulse rate and quality.

    B. SAMPLE history.

    C. airway and breathing status.

    D. skin color and temperature.

44. Which of the following is **not** a link in the American Heart Association's chain of survival?

    A. early access

    B. early CPR

    C. early diagnosis

    D. early defibrillation

45. Which of the following statements is **incorrect** pertaining to ventricular fibrillation and defibrillation?

    A. Ventricular fibrillation is the most common initial rhythm in sudden cardiac arrest.

    B. Early CPR and electrical defibrillation is the most successful treatment for ventricular fibrillation.

    C. When CPR is performed, successful defibrillation time may be extended.

    D. Ventricular fibrillation will last long periods of time before deteriorating to asystole.

46. You have delivered a shock using a semi-automated AED. The AED gives a "No Shock" message. Your next action should be:
    A. check the patient's pulse.
    B. deliver the third shock.
    C. reposition the adhesive pads.
    D. begin CPR immediately.

47. Why must CPR be stopped while the AED is analyzing the rhythm?
    A. The device emits oral messages that may **not** be heard during CPR.
    B. The device senses the CPR compressions and cannot be turned on.
    C. The device may automatically deliver a shock.
    D. The device cannot analyze the rhythm while CPR is being performed.

48. While the AED is performing its analysis before shock is delivered, you should:
    A. perform CPR.
    B. auscultate breath sounds.
    C. check for a carotid pulse.
    D. remain clear of the patient.

49. You have provided one shock with the AED. The patient has regained a pulse. Your next immediate action should be:
    A. assess the blood pressure.
    B. check the patient's breathing.
    C. perform a focused history.
    D. provide advanced cardiac life support (ACLS) immediately.

50. It is questionable to use an AED for children under what age?
    A. 12
    B. 10
    C. 8
    D. 1

51. Patients who complain of chest pain:
    A. require the application and use of the AED.
    B. require the AED only if in respiratory arrest.
    C. may deteriorate to cardiac arrest.
    D. will go into cardiac arrest within 1 hour.

52. Defibrillation is most successful for patients in cardiac arrest resulting from:
    A. stroke.
    B. hypoglycemia.
    C. a dysrhythmia associated with coronary artery disease.
    D. an auto accident involving head trauma and hypoventilation for the patient.

53. Which of the following sign(s) of cardiac arrest must be present in order to attach the AED to the patient?
    A. no pulse and dilated pupils
    B. no respirations and no spontaneous movement
    C. unresponsive only
    D. no pulse, unresponsive, and no respirations

54. The patient you are treating suddenly grabs his chest and closes his eyes. He is unresponsive to pain and verbal stimuli and is pulseless and breathless. You place the patient on the AED and analyze the rhythm. The AED advises "No Shock." You should next:
    A. check the breathing.
    B. begin chest compressions.
    C. check the patient's pulse.
    D. re-analyze the rhythm.

55. After your analysis of the rhythm, the AED advises "Deliver Shock." It is important to:
    A. check the patient's pulse before delivering the shock.
    B. check with medical control before delivering the shock.
    C. ensure that all personnel are clear of the patient.
    D. ventilate twice before delivering the shock.

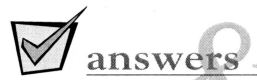

answers & rationales

Following each rationale, you will find a reference to the corresponding D.O.T. objective. A rationale marked with an asterisk denotes material supplemental to the First Responder curriculum. Also included after each rationale are references to where the question topic may be covered in Brady First Responder textbooks. **"FR7" refers to *First Responder, 7e*** (Bergeron, Bizjak, Krause, Le Baudour). **"FRASA" refers to *First Responder: A Skills Approach, 7e*** (Limmer, Karren, Hafen).

1.

C. The most common cause of cardiac arrest is related to heart disease. Coronary artery disease is likely the contributing factor to either a heart attack or cardiac rhythm disturbance that leads to cardiac arrest. (4-1.1) (FR7 p. 185; FRASA p. 148)

2.

D. The most common cause of cardiac arrest in infants and young children is airway obstruction or a breathing disturbance. Either an airway disturbance or breathing problem will lead to severe hypoxia (low oxygen level), causing the heart to stop. (4-1.1) (FR7 p. 108; FRASA p. 158)

3.

A. Cardiopulmonary resuscitation is composed of establishing unresponsiveness, opening the airway, assessing breathing, administering positive pressure ventilation, assessing circulation, and performing chest compressions. Administration of medications is part of advanced cardiac life support and not basic CPR. (4-1.2) (FR7 pp. 185–186; FRASA pp. 150–152)

4.

A. The first link in the chain of survival is to access EMS. This is typically done most quickly by dialing 911. The second link is to perform cardiopulmonary resuscitation followed by early defibrillation. The last link is provision of advanced life support. (4-1.3) (FR7 p. 184; FRASA p. 148–149)

5.

C. Blood is pumped from the right atrium to the right ventricle to the lungs back to the left atrium to the left ventricle and through the aorta and finally to the body. (4-1.2) (FR7 pp. 284–285; FRASA p. 147)

6.

B. Oxygen, carbon dioxide, and other nutrients are exchanged in the capillaries. (4-1.2) (FR7 p. 100; FRASA p. 58)

7.

C. The right side of the heart is a low-pressure pump that pumps the blood to the lungs and then to the high-pressure left side that pumps the blood to the body. (4-1.2) (FR7 pp. 284–285; FRASA pp. 147–148)

8.

C. The first step in caring for this patient would be to establish unresponsiveness. (4-1.4) (FR7 p. 185; FRASA p. 149)

9.

A. The next step in the sequence is to open the airway and then assess for breathing. (4-1.4) (FR7 p. 185; FRASA p. 149)

10.

B. The carotid pulse should be checked on the unresponsive patient, especially if suspected of being in cardiac arrest. A brachial pulse will be the preferred pulse to check on an infant (less than 1 year of age). (4-1.4) (FR7 p. 187; FRASA pp. 149, 161)

11.

B. While performing one- or two-person CPR on an adult when the airway is not protected, 30 compressions should be delivered followed by two ventilations. (4-1.4) (FR7 p. 191; FRASA pp. 152, 155)

12.

C. The compression rate for one- or two-person CPR is approximately 100 compressions per minute. (4-1.4) (FR7 p. 192; FRASA p. 152)

13.

C. When providing ventilation to a patient, it is essential to deliver supplemental oxygen via the ventilation device as quickly as possible. If oxygen is not being delivered, or if the concentration being delivered is less than 40 percent, you must deliver a higher tidal volume (10 ml/kg) with each breath. After oxygen is connected and is being delivered at a concentration of greater than 400 percent, the tidal volume can be reduced to 6–7 ml/kg. The increase in oxygen delivered allows for the reduction in volume delivered. (4-1.4)

14.

B. When performing chest compressions on an adult patient, you should compress the chest $1\frac{1}{2}$–2 inches. If that does not produce palpable pulses with each compression, the depth of compression should be adjusted until pulses are palpated. (4-1.5) (FR7 p. 190; FRASA p. 152). Remember that compressions should be hard and fast at a rate of 100/minute.

15.

C. The landmark for infant chest compression is two fingers placed one finger's width below the intermammary line. (4-1.6) (FR7 p. 214; FRASA pp. 160–161)

16.

D. A 5-year-old is considered a child for the purposes of CPR. The heel of one or two hands should be placed on the lower half of the sternum and the chest compressed one-third to one-half the depth of the chest. (4-1.11) (FR7 p. 213; FRASA pp. 160, 163)

17.

C. In the child, 30 compressions should be delivered followed by 2 ventilations. (4-1.7) (FR7 p. 214; FRASA pp. 160, 163)

18.

B. Upon entry of the second rescuer, he or she should immediately assess for effectiveness of compressions by checking the carotid pulse. Once the compressor has finished the cycle, check for pulse and breathing and then continue with two-person CPR. (4-1.9) (FR7 p. 197; FRASA p. 155) At a rate of 30–2 the second rescuer takes over compressions.

19.

C. Ventilations in the infant and child should be delivered over 1 second. This helps reduce the incidence of gastric inflation and regurgitation. (4-1.11) (FR7 p. 105; FRASA p. 109)

20.

C. It is acceptable to stop compressions once the EMS crew has arrived and you have been instructed to do so. (4-1.8) (FR7 p. 222; FRASA p. 149)

21.

D. The AED should only be applied to patients older than 1 year of age who are unresponsive, pulseless, and apneic where the cardiac arrest is not due primarily to a traumatic incident. If the AED is applied to a preadolescent child, it is strongly recommended that pediatric AED pads be used. These pads are designed to reduce the energy flow through a resistor so that a smaller amount of energy is delivered to the child. If no pediatric AED pads are available, as a last resort, the adult pads can be applied to the child. (*) (FR7 p. 206; FRASA p. 169)

22.

C. A patient who is having difficulty breathing or who is suffering from congestive heart failure should be placed in a position of comfort, which is most likely with the head and chest in an upright and elevated position. (*) (FR7 p. 238; FRASA p. 257)

23.

C. Ventricular fibrillation is the most common presenting rhythm in the first 8 minutes of cardiac arrest. (*) (FR7 p. 204; FRASA p. 169)

24.

C. The most effective treatment of ventricular fibrillation in an unwitnessed arrest is 2 minutes of CPR followed by defibrillation. (*) (FRASA pp. 170, 173)

25.

C. When you are a single rescuer, you should deliver one shock and then leave to activate the EMS system. This allows for early defibrillation and early access to ALS care. (*) (FR7 p. 208; FRASA p. 173)

26.

C. Defibrillation has already been proven to be the most effective treatment for ventricular fibrillation. Reducing the time to defibrillation and good CPR, working with ALS units more effectively, and determining if further training is needed are aspects that can be reviewed. (*) (FR7 p. 210; FRASA p. 173)

27.

A. If you are trained and proficient in the use of the AED, the first defibrillation in a witnessed arrest can be administered within 1 minute of the arrival of the AED at the patient's side. Once the patient has been determined to be pulseless, defibrillation takes precedence over all other assessments and treatments. (*) (FRASA pp. 169–170)

28.

D. Weak or dead batteries are the most common cause of failure of the AED. Because of this, it is imperative to check the batteries each and every shift. (*) (FRASA p. 173)

29.

C. The completion of the checklist assures you that the machine is in working order. What it does not ensure is that the operator is proficient in the use of the AED. (*) (FR7 p. 211)

30.

D. Studies have shown that to be most effective the defibrillation should occur within 4 minutes. (*) (FRASA p. 170)

31.

A. The studies have proven that if bystander CPR is started immediately, defibrillation can be successful for up to 10 minutes after cardiac arrest. (*) (FR7 p. 186; FRASA p. 148)

32.

D. You should minimize interruptions in compressions when performing CPR. After defibrillation, a pulse check will be done after 5 cycles, approximately 2 minutes, of CPR. (*) (FR7 p. 208; FRASA p. 171)

33.

C. Proper CPR requires full chest recoil after each compression. To achieve full recoil, you must bring your hands up fully after each compression. The chest should return to its normal position. Complete recoil allows maximum return of blood to the heart after each compression. Compressions should be hard and fast. (*) (FR7 p. 191; FRASA p. 152)

34.

C. The AED should be placed only on an unresponsive, pulseless, apneic patient. (*) (FR7 p. 206; FRASA p. 167)

35.

B. If the patient becomes pulseless and apneic, you should immediately analyze the rhythm and deliver a shock if it is indicated. (*) (FR7 pp. 208–209; FRASA p. 173)

36.

B. If a patient regains a pulse and then loses it again, you should proceed with immediate defibrillation; only one defibrillation is delivered. (*) (FR7 p. 208; FRASA p. 173)

37.

C. The post-resuscitation patient should be reassessed at least every 5 minutes or whenever the patient's condition changes. (*) (FR7 p. 210; FRASA pp. 173, 229)

38.

C. Whenever the AED advises "No Shock," you should perform CPR for 2 minutes, reassess for a pulse and then re-analyze the rhythm. (4-3.25) (FR7 p. 210; FRASA p. 173)

39.

B. Currently there is not enough evidence to recommend for or against the use of AEDs in infants less than 1 year of age. It is acceptable to apply and use the device on a patient who is elderly or who recently had open-heart surgery. (*) (FR7 p. 206; FRASA p. 169)

40.

B. All patients who complain of chest pain or discomfort should receive oxygen at 15 lpm by nonrebreather mask. Chest pain or discomfort is commonly caused by the lack of oxygen to the cardiac tissue. When cardiac tissue becomes inadequately oxygenated, the area affected becomes hypoxic, stimulating the pain.

High-flow oxygen can help reduce damage to the cardiac tissue and potentially reduce the size of the heart attack. (*) (FR7 p. 235; FRASA p. 129, 252)

41.

D. First perform a general impression and assess the mental status. You must then ensure an adequate airway. Next, assess the breathing for adequacy. Determine if the patient is breathing normally or with increased effort. Following the breathing assessment, check the pulse. Is circulation adequate? Finally, assess the skin. Is the patient pale, cyanotic, cool, clammy? This quick assessment will help you to rapidly determine the patient's condition. (*) (FR7 pp. 233–235; FRASA pp. 216–220)

42.

A. Approximately 20 percent of heart attacks are silent. There is no chest pain associated with the event. Silent heart attacks occur more frequently in the elderly because of diminished sensation of pain. Other assessment findings such as shortness of breath, nausea, vomiting, anxiety, abnormal blood pressure, abnormal pulse, dizziness, and feeling of impending doom should raise your suspicion of a silent heart attack. (*) (FRASA p. 255)

43.

C. Your first concern is to ensure the patient has an adequate airway. You should then assess the breathing and circulation. It is crucial to provide positive pressure ventilation if the ventilation status is inadequate. Early recognition and treatment of the patient with cardiac compromise will help increase the patient's survival. (*) (FR7 pp. 232–234; FRASA p. 252)

44.

C. Early diagnosis is not a part of the chain of survival. Early access is crucial. The sooner CPR is provided, the greater the chances of survival. Early defibrillation may restore a functional heartbeat to the patient, thus providing better circulation of oxygen. Early ALS will provide medications and other techniques that increase the survival of the patient and reduce the chance of the patient refibrillating. (*) (FR7 p. 184; FRASA pp. 148–149)

45.

D. Ventricular fibrillation quickly deteriorates into asystole (no electrical activity in the heart or "flat line"). The most effective defibrillation with successful conversion typically occurs within 4 minutes of the onset of cardiac arrest. As time elapses without defibrillation, the success rate falls significantly. In an unwitnessed arrest that is greater than 4 to 5 minutes, it is necessary to perform 2 minutes of CPR prior to defibrillation. (*) (FR7 p. 204; FRASA p. 169)

46.

D. When the AED delivers a shock and then gives a "No Shock" message, you will begin chest compressions immediately. (*) (FR7 pp. 209–210; FRASA pp. 171–172)

47.

D. The AED cannot effectively analyze the rhythm during CPR. The compression of the heart muscle produces electrical activity that produces artifact. The AED reads this rhythm and is unable to determine if a shock is needed. (*) (FR7 p. 210; FRASA pp. 171–172)

48.

D. The AED is a sensitive device that can be influenced by outside interference. When the AED is performing an analysis of the patient, you should not touch the patient. Touching the patient may interfere with the analysis. (*) (FR7 p. 208; FRASA p. 171)

49.

B. Your next action after checking the pulse following successful defibrillation is to assess the patient's breathing. If breathing is adequate, provide oxygen at 15 lpm via nonrebreather mask. If the breathing is inadequate, provide positive pressure ventilation with supplemental oxygen. (*) (FR7 p. 208; FRASA p. 171)

50.

D. Currently there is not enough evidence to recommend for or against the use of AEDs in infants less than 1 year of age. For pediatric patients, it is preferable to use an AED with pediatric pads that allow for a reduced energy delivery. However, if only an adult AED is available, it may be used on a pediatric patient who is in cardiac arrest and more than 1 year of age. (*) (FR7 p. 206; FRASA p. 169)

51.

C. Not all patients with chest pain or cardiac compromise will go into cardiac arrest. Monitor the chest pain patient closely. If the patient becomes unresponsive, pulseless, and breathless, application of the AED is indicated. (*) (FR7 p. 231; FRASA p. 252)

52.

C. Defibrillation or the use of the AED is most useful for patients in cardiac arrest resulting from dysrhythmias associated with coronary artery disease. The other patients have etiologies of cardiac arrest that require alternative management. (*) (FR7 p. 203; FRASA p. 169)

53.

D. All three signs of cardiac arrest must be present to apply the AED: no respirations, no pulse, and the patient must not respond to verbal or pain stimuli (unresponsive). (*) (FR7 p. 206; FRASA p. 149)

54.

B. If the AED advises "No Shock," immediately begin chest compressions for 2 minutes and then check pulse and re-analyze the rhythm. (*) (FR7 pp. 209–210; FRASA p. 171)

55.

C. Before delivery of the shock, ensure that rescuers and bystanders are all clear of the patient and that no one is in contact with the patient. (*) (FR7 p. 208; FRASA pp. 171–173)

5 Illness and Injury

module objectives

Questions in this module relate to D.O.T.
objectives 5-1.1 to 5-3.8.

DIRECTIONS Each of the questions or incomplete statements below is followed by suggested answers or completions. Select the **one answer** that is best in each case.

MEDICAL EMERGENCIES 5-1

Altered Mental Status and Diabetic Emergencies

1. You arrive on-scene to find the apartment manager urging you to come inside. You survey the scene and find no immediate dangers, so you proceed in. The manager tells you that he brought the patient his evening meal and found him on the floor unresponsive. You assess the patient, and your partner begins to look around the apartment for any further clues. Your assessment reveals a male patient unresponsive to verbal stimuli, blood pressure 120/68, pulse rate 122, respiratory rate 18, and cool, moist skin. Your partner comes back with a pill bottle of Micronase he found on the counter. From your assessment findings and the patient's medication, you suspect he is most likely suffering from:
   A. a myocardial infarction.
   B. a stroke.
   C. low blood sugar level (hypoglycemia).
   D. high blood sugar level (hyperglycemia).

2. Which of the following signs or symptoms would most likely indicate the patient is suffering from a low blood sugar level in a diabetic patient?
   A. very rapid onset of an altered mental status
   B. tachycardia
   C. cool, moist skin
   D. all of the above

3. In order to administer instant glucose or any sugar solution by mouth, a patient must have:
   A. an intact gag reflex and an ability to swallow.
   B. a history of diabetic seizures.

   C. a history of epilepsy controlled by medications.
   D. an altered mental status with only a response to painful stimuli.

4. The proper administration of instant glucose includes:
   A. allowing the patient to suck on the tube until the symptoms appear to resolve.
   B. placing a pinch between the patient's cheek and gum every 3–5 minutes until the symptoms resolve.
   C. placing the glucose on a tongue depressor, placing the depressor between the cheek and gum, and rubbing the area.
   D. squirting approximately half the tube into the patient's mouth and allowing it to dissolve.

5. Your patient is suffering from an altered mental status. The patient has a history of diabetes that is controlled with medication. The patient, however, has snoring respirations and is responsive only to painful stimuli. You should:
   A. open the airway and place a pinch of glucose between his cheek and gum.
   B. open the airway, place a small amount of glucose on a tongue depressor, and place it between the gum and cheek.
   C. open the patient's airway and call for immediate transport.
   D. open the patient's airway, insert an airway adjunct, and continue your assessment.

6. A contraindication to the administration of oral glucose or a high sugar solution by mouth in a diabetic patient is:
   A. inability to swallow or unconsciousness.
   B. decreased level of consciousness.
   C. heart rate greater than 100 bpm.
   D. headache and sweating.

7. Your patient has a history of diabetes that is controlled by medication. The patient is unresponsive to verbal stimuli but responds to pain. Which of the following emergency care is most appropriate?
   A. place the patient in a Trendelenburg (shock) position and administer oral glucose
   B. administer oral glucose or a glucose solution and position on his side
   C. maintain an open airway and place the patient in a Fowler (sitting) position
   D. maintain open airway and position on his side

8. While you are administering oral glucose to an insulin-dependent diabetic patient, the patient becomes unresponsive. You should immediately:
   A. reassess the patient's airway, breathing, and circulation status.
   B. place the patient in a semi-sitting position.
   C. try to remove the drug by gently scraping the cheek.
   D. administer an additional dose to quickly raise the blood glucose level.

9. A priority in managing the patient with an altered mental status is:
   A. the administration of oral glucose.
   B. maintenance of a patent airway.
   C. obtaining an accurate and complete history.
   D. completion of an early detailed physical exam.

10. Place the following treatment steps for the patient with an altered mental status in the most appropriate order:

   1. Insert an oropharyngeal or nasopharyngeal airway.
   2. Suction secretions.
   3. Manually open the airway.
   4. Position the patient in a left lateral recumbent position.

   A. 1, 2, 4, 3
   B. 4, 2, 1, 3
   C. 2, 4, 1, 3
   D. 3, 2, 1, 4

11. You are managing a patient who has an altered mental status. During your assessment and treatment you must:
   A. place the patient in a supine (face-up) position.
   B. administer a solution containing glucose.
   C. explain everything you are doing to the patient.
   D. place the patient in a prone (face-down) position .

ALTERED MENTAL STATUS—STROKE

12. A sign of a stroke may include which of the following?
   A. aphasia (cannot speak)
   B. hemiplegia (paralysis to one side of the body)
   C. hemiparesis (weakness to one side of the body)
   D. all of the above

13. The difference between a stroke and a TIA (transient ischemic attack) is:
   A. a TIA usually only involves one side of the body while a stroke affects both sides.
   B. a stroke usually causes a TIA.
   C. the signs and symptoms of a TIA disappear within 24 hours and usually result in no permanent neurological dysfunction.
   D. only patients suffering a stroke require transport and treatment.

14. You arrive on-scene and find your patient supine (face-up) on the floor. The patient's wife tells you that he just got back from running and complained of "the worst headache of my life" and then fell to the ground. You suspect the patient has suffered from which of the following illnesses?
    A. heart attack
    B. hemorrhagic stroke
    C. allergic reaction
    D. transient ischemic attack

15. Which of the following may be a late sign or symptom of a stroke?
    A. unequal pupils
    B. headache
    C. seizures
    D. stiff neck

16. Which of the following is **not** a common sign or symptom of a stroke?
    A. loss of bowel and bladder control
    B. hemiplegia (paralysis to one side of the body)
    C. severe intermittent abdominal pain
    D. unequal pupils with loss of vision in one eye

17. Your patient awoke this morning and felt dizzy. He also experienced nausea with vomiting. You note incomprehensible speech and unequal pupils. You suspect:
    A. heart attack.
    B. stroke.
    C. low blood sugar level.
    D. seizure disorder.

ALTERED MENTAL STATUS— POISONING/OVERDOSE

18. All of the following may be signs and symptoms of a poisoning except:
    A. severe headache.
    B. unequal pupils.
    C. slow heart rate.
    D. abdominal pain.

19. Your first priority in providing emergency medical care to a patient who has overdosed on an unknown medication is:
    A. administering activated charcoal.
    B. identifying the medication taken.
    C. administering high-flow oxygen.
    D. maintaining a patent airway.

20. While you are transporting a patient who has overdosed on sleeping pills, the respiratory rate decreases from 20 to 8 times a minute. Your immediate action should be to:
    A. administer activated charcoal.
    B. provide positive pressure ventilation.
    C. administer oxygen by nonrebreather mask.
    D. position the patient in the Trendelenburg position.

21. In which of the following poisoned patients is activated charcoal indicated?
    A. 8-year-old who mistakenly drank liquid bleach less than 1 hour ago
    B. 38-year-old who has inhaled carbon monoxide 3 hours ago
    C. 60-year-old who has overdosed on blood pressure pills 2 hours ago
    D. 3-year-old who has ingested liquid ammonia less than 10 minutes ago

22. Activated charcoal:
    A. increases urinary output, which forcefully eliminates the poison.
    B. speeds absorption into the body where it is eliminated quickly.
    C. adsorbs the contaminant, inhibiting absorption into the body.
    D. actively neutralizes most poisons, rendering them harmless.

23. Poisons may enter the body by:
    A. ingestion.
    B. inhalation.
    C. injection.
    D. all of the above.

24. You are assisting a patient who is having chest pain and takes a nitroglycerin tablet by placing it under the tongue. This is an example of what type of route the medication uses to enter the body?
    A. inhalation
    B. ingestion
    C. absorption
    D. injection

25. A patient is suffering an anaphylactic reaction from a yellow jacket bite. By what route did the venom enter the patient's body?
    A. absorption
    B. injection
    C. inhalation
    D. ingestion

26. Emergency care for a dry powder absorption poison would include:
    A. covering the patient's arm with a burn sheet to preserve the powder for the emergency room.
    B. immediately washing the powder off to prevent further exposure.
    C. brushing the powder off before irrigating the contaminated area.
    D. flushing the area with water and then brushing the area dry.

27. You are called to the scene for a possible chlorine leak. As you pull up to the scene, you see two victims lying on the ground by a tool shed. Your immediate action(s) include:
    A. removing the victims from the scene to prevent further injury.
    B. immediately providing positive pressure ventilation to the victims to prevent further hypoxia.

    C. rapidly extricating the patients from the chlorine gas.
    D. immediately moving to a safe environment uphill and upwind and contacting the fire department.

28. What position should you place the medical patient in to prevent aspiration?
    A. prone
    B. lateral recumbent
    C. Fowler's
    D. supine

29. In cases of poisoning, your best resource for information regarding treatment of the patient is:
    A. the patient's family physician.
    B. drug/chemical information booklet.
    C. poison control center.
    D. handheld drug reference.

30. Your patient has swallowed industrial drain cleaner in a possible suicide attempt. She responds only to deep painful stimuli and is breathing 6 times per minute. Your treatment for this patient would include all of the following **except:**
    A. maintaining a patent airway.
    B. flushing the mouth to remove any cleaner to prevent further contamination.
    C. providing positive pressure ventilation.
    D. inserting a nasopharyngeal airway.

31. Activated charcoal is only indicated for poisoning that occurs by:
    A. ingestion.
    B. injection.
    C. absorption.
    D. inhalation.

32. Which of the following is **not** a contraindication for the use of activated charcoal?
    A. The patient is unable to swallow.
    B. The patient has ingested ammonia.
    C. The patient is fully alert.
    D. The patient has ingested bleach.

33. Which of the following does **not** indicate an emergency that is due to drugs or alcohol?
    A. empty liquor bottles
    B. hospital discharge orders
    C. home oxygen unit
    D. prescription bottles

34. The "Talk-Down Technique" for managing a violent drug or alcohol patient is not useful for patients who have taken:
    A. phencyclidine.
    B. cocaine.
    C. crack.
    D. marijuana.

SEIZURES

35. A sudden and temporary alteration in behavior caused by the massive electrical discharge from a neuron or group of neurons in the brain is a:
    A. stroke.
    B. seizure.
    C. TIA.
    D. cerebral hemorrhage.

36. The pattern or sequence of events for a generalized tonic-clonic seizure includes:
    A. seizure, aura, postictal state.
    B. aura, clonic phase, tonic phase, postictal state.
    C. aura, tonic phase, myotonic phase, postictal state.
    D. aura, tonic phase, clonic phase, postictal state.

37. Which of the following are possible causes of seizures?
    A. infection
    B. high fever
    C. hypoxia
    D. all of the above

38. Treatment for a patient who is actively seizing includes:
    A. protecting and positioning the patient, maintaining an airway, administering oral glucose or a glucose solution, suctioning the airway, and applying supplemental oxygen.
    B. protecting and positioning the patient, prying the mouth open to insert an oral airway, suctioning the airway, applying supplemental oxygen, and calling for rapid transport.
    C. protecting and positioning the patient, maintaining an airway, suctioning the airway, assisting ventilations if necessary, and applying supplemental oxygen.
    D. protecting and positioning the patient, maintaining an airway, suctioning the airway, assisting ventilations if needed, applying supplemental oxygen, and waiting for the patient to regain consciousness to sign a refusal form.

39. A patient having seizures lasting more than 5 minutes or seizures that occur without a period of consciousness between is considered to be suffering from:
    A. a grand mal seizure.
    B. tonic-clonic seizures.
    C. status epilepticus.
    D. a prolonged hysterical seizure.

40. The preferred airway adjunct for an actively seizing patient with clenched teeth is the:
    A. nasopharyngeal airway.
    B. oropharyngeal airway.
    C. tracheal tube.
    D. combitube.

41. A patient who suffers two or more consecutive seizures without a period of consciousness between them or a seizure that lasts longer than 5 minutes has a condition referred to as:
    A. continual epilepsy.
    B. continual seizure.
    C. status epilepticus.
    D. status seizure.

42. The patient with a history of epilepsy suddenly states she is experiencing a metallic taste in her mouth. She says it is an aura. She will next likely suffer:

    A. a postictal state.

    B. a petit mal seizure.

    C. a generalized tonic-clonic seizure.

    D. a focal motor seizure.

43. Which stage of a seizure is known as the recovery phase during which the patient's mental status progressively improves over time?

    A. postictal phase

    B. tonic phase

    C. clonic phase

    D. aura phase

44. A syncopal episode usually begins while the patient is in which position?

    A. lying

    B. kneeling

    C. standing

    D. sitting

45. You are treating a patient who has experienced a syncopal episode. You should place this patient in which position?

    A. sitting with head between the knees

    B. supine with the legs elevated

    C. prone with the head elevated

    D. Fowler with the feet elevated

46. A bystander states your patient was standing when he became dizzy and then unresponsive. After the patient was assisted to the floor, he immediately became responsive again. The skin is pale and moist. You suspect:

    A. a generalized seizure.

    B. a syncopal episode.

C. a heart attack.

D. hypoglycemia.

47. A febrile seizure would be considered serious if it lasted longer than:

    A. 3 minutes.

    B. 5 minutes.

    C. 10 minutes.

    D. 15 minutes.

ENVIRONMENTAL—HEAT AND COLD EMERGENCIES

48. What is the most significant mechanism of heat loss (approximately 60 percent) that involves the transfer of heat from the surface of one object to another without physical contact?

    A. convection

    B. conduction

    C. evaporation

    D. radiation

49. Taking into consideration the process of conduction and water chill, how much faster than any other mechanism will wet clothing conduct heat away from the body?

    A. 100 times faster

    B. 200 times faster

    C. 240 times faster

    D. 275 times faster

50. All of the following are early signs of hypothermia (cold exposure) except:

    A. muscle stiffness.

    B. slow heart rate.

    C. uncoordination.

    D. rapid heart rate.

51. When a patient is surrounded by water that has the same temperature as that of the ambient air:

    A. the core temperature will drop 25–30 times faster in the water than in the ambient air.

    B. the core temperature will stay the same as the temperature of the ambient air regardless of the temperature of the water.

    C. the core temperature will drop 100 times faster in the water than in the ambient air.

    D. the core temperature will not drop as fast because the water will act as an insulator of body heat.

52. Characteristics that predispose the elderly to heat emergencies include:

    A. poor thermoregulation.

    B. the tendency for the elderly to retire to communities in hotter climates.

    C. poor fluid intake and hydration status.

    D. all of the above.

53. Treatment for a patient suffering from a heat emergency with hot dry skin includes all of the following **except:**

    A. removing the patient from the hot environment.

    B. cooling the patient with cool water, ice packs, and fans.

    C. administration of high-flow oxygen.

    D. covering the patient with blankets to prevent cooling too rapidly.

54. Infants and young children lose heat more quickly than adults do because:

    A. they are smaller in size with a larger surface area.

    B. they cannot protect themselves from temperature changes by putting on or taking off their clothes.

    C. they usually have proportionately less body fat than adults.

    D. all of the above.

55. Which of the following is an appropriate treatment for the patient with generalized hypothermia?

    A. Transfer, move, or handle the patient as you would any other patient.

    B. Provide CPR and defibrillate as needed if the patient is in cardiac arrest.

    C. Rub or massage the patient's arms or legs.

    D. Hyperventilate the patient at a rate of 24 breaths per minute.

56. When managing a hypothermic patient, you cannot detect a pulse or respiration, but the patient moves; you should:

    A. start CPR immediately.

    B. start CPR and apply the AED immediately.

    C. begin positive pressure ventilation.

    D. apply the AED to determine the patient's rhythm.

57. Which of the following is appropriate management for a patient with immersion hypothermia?

    A. Instruct the patient to swim and tread water as vigorously as possible.

    B. Lift the patient from the water in a horizontal position.

    C. Lift the patient from the water in a vertical position.

    D. Leave the wet clothing on the patient to insulate him or her from heat loss upon removal from the water.

58. Appropriate emergency management of a localized cold injury includes:

    A. massaging the affected skin.

    B. removing jewelry.

    C. applying of a salve or ointment to open wounds.

    D. breaking blisters that are present on the surface of the skin.

59. Rewarming of localized frozen tissue:
    A. is safe to perform on all patients.
    B. can be safely performed by using dry heat.
    C. requires water of 120–130° F.
    D. is extremely painful for the patient.

SCENARIO

Questions 60–62 refer to the following scenario:

It is midsummer and you have been dispatched to a local park for a man down. You arrive and observe a workman who appears to be in his 40s lying supine. He is in the full sun and is next to a ditch. A coworker informs you that the patient was digging the ditch and just passed out. The patient's eyes are closed, and he does not respond to your voice or painful stimuli. His respirations are deep and rapid. His pulse is 110 bpm, regular, and strong. His skin is hot and slightly moist. The coworker further informs you that the patient had complained of a headache and nausea for at least 30 minutes prior to passing out.

60. Which action should be taken first?
    A. Administer oxygen at 15 lpm.
    B. Apply cold packs to the patient's body.
    C. Remove the patient's clothing.
    D. Move the patient to a cooler environment.

61. This patient is considered:
    A. a high priority.
    B. a medium priority.
    C. a low priority.
    D. a patient not requiring additional care or transport.

62. The patient is most likely suffering from a _____. This is common on days when the temperature is greater than _____ °F with a relative humidity greater than _____ percent.
    A. vascular accident, 80, 90
    B. heat seizure, 80, 65
    C. heat emergency, 80, 65
    D. heat emergency, 90, 75

63. Which of the following is **not** a predisposing factor that increases the risk of hypothermia (cold emergency)?
    A. alcohol use
    B. family history
    C. medical conditions
    D. patient's age

64. The first compensatory mechanism the body uses to try to maintain body temperature in a cold emergency is:
    A. increased heart rate.
    B. increased respirations.
    C. shivering and goose bumps.
    D. increased fine-motor function.

65. You are treating a responsive patient who is experiencing a heat emergency. The patient's skin is moist, pale, and cool. Which treatment is incorrect for this patient?
    A. Have the patient drink cool water if not nauseated.
    B. Place the patient in a seated position.
    C. Cool the patient with wet compresses.
    D. Administer oxygen by nonrebreather mask at 15 lpm if allowed by protocol.

BEHAVIORAL AND PSYCHOLOGICAL CRISIS

66. The manner in which a person acts, including any and all physical and mental activity, is a definition of:
    A. anxiety.
    B. behavior.
    C. depression.
    D. morals and ethics.

67. A behavioral emergency is best defined as:

    A. behavior that is unethical.

    B. behavior that does not represent what the prudent person would do in certain situations.

    C. behavior that is "abnormal" in the given situation and intolerable to the patient, community, or family.

    D. any situation that requires a psychiatric consultation.

68. A patient thought to be suffering from a behavioral emergency might be actually suffering from:

    A. hypoglycemia (low blood sugar level).

    B. hypoxia (low oxygen level).

    C. head injury.

    D. all of the above.

69. You are called to the scene for a patient who was struck by an automobile. There are no witnesses, and the driver states that the patient came out of nowhere. While on the scene, the patient states that all he wanted to do was to die. Your reaction to this comment should be to:

    A. assume the patient has suffered severe head trauma and is incoherent.

    B. assume the patient is intoxicated and doesn't know what he is saying.

    C. pay no attention to the remark because the patient may be delirious from the accident or suffering a head injury.

    D. report the statement to the EMS crew because the accident may have been a suicide attempt.

70. Risk factors that are suggestive of suicidal tendencies include:

    A. recent marriage.

    B. ages of 17 through 30.

    C. loss of a significant loved one.

    D. recent promotion with additional stress.

71. What percentage of patients who succeed in committing suicide have made previous attempts?

    A. approximately 90 percent

    B. approximately 80 percent

    C. approximately 50 percent

    D. approximately 40 percent

72. During the assessment of a despondent patient, you notice multiple cuts on the victim's wrists and arms. You should be concerned that the patient:

    A. may have been involved in a fight.

    B. may have been tied up for a period of time.

    C. may have attempted suicide.

    D. is an IV drug user and possibly HIV positive.

73. When determining suicidal tendencies, the patient most likely to commit suicide is one who:

    A. has been drinking heavily and is depressed.

    B. has a definite suicide plan.

    C. has a history of drug abuse.

    D. is middle-aged and suffering from a chronic disease.

74. When a patient tells you that he or she has thought of harming himself or herself with a gun, you should:

    A. do nothing because this is just a way to gain attention.

    B. make sure that the patient is not armed and is of no danger to you.

    C. ask the patient to show you the gun, as this will prove his or her intentions.

    D. attempt to console the patient and find out why the patient wants to hurt himself or herself.

75. You are called to a private residence for an unknown emergency. You walk into the residence and find an elderly man sitting among bottles of whiskey, crying over a picture. You observe a pistol in the patient's waistband. Your first action should be to:

    A. ask the patient why he is so sad.

    B. determine if the patient wants to kill himself.

    C. slowly and calmly back out of the room.

    D. charge the patient and pin him down.

76. In the previous patient, all of the following are risk factors of suicide except:

    A. the patient sitting amongst whiskey bottles, possibly indicating a substance abuse problem.

    B. the patient's age. Older individuals usually are more mature and less likely to commit suicide.

    C. the patient's sex. Males are more likely to commit suicide than are females.

    D. the patient's firearm.

77. When assessing a patient whom you believe is a risk for violence, you should:

    A. assess the patient with adequate help to restrain the patient if he or she becomes violent.

    B. make sure that all potential weapons or unsafe objects are out of his or her reach.

    C. ask the patient if he or she wants to kill himself or herself.

    D. all of the above.

78. Which of the following can cause a patient to exhibit signs of aggression?

    A. fear

    B. anxiety

    C. hypoglycemia (low blood sugar level)

    D. all of the above

79. When asking a patient about suicidal intentions, you should do all of the following except:

    A. remain nonjudgmental.

    B. explain to the patient that his or her thoughts are irrational.

    C. ask the patient if he or she wants to kill himself or herself.

    D. be honest at all times.

80. You have restrained a patient who was exhibiting violent behavior toward his family. After a period of time, the patient calms down and wants the restraints removed. You should:

    A. remove the restraints if the patient states he is no longer violent.

    B. not remove the restraints for the safety of you, your crew, and the patient.

    C. remove the leg restraints only and see how the patient responds.

    D. remove the wrist restraints only for a short time and monitor the patient's behavior.

ENRICHMENT

Respiratory

81. Components of the respiratory system include all of the following except:

    A. lung.

    B. larynx.

    C. esophagus.

    D. trachea.

82. Which of the following are functions of the nose?

    A. warm inspired air

    B. filter out large dust particles

    C. humidify inspired air

    D. all of the above

83. Which structure is responsible for controlling the movement of food and air between the respiratory and digestive systems?
    A. pharynx
    B. epiglottis
    C. thyroid cartilage
    D. cricoid cartilage

84. The major muscle of respiration is the:
    A. external intercostal muscle.
    B. internal intercostal muscle.
    C. diaphragm.
    D. pectoralis major.

85. Which of the following is an early sign of hypoxia?
    A. red warm skin
    B. tachycardia
    C. bradycardia
    D. all of the above

86. To determine if the patient has adequate breathing, the First Responder should do all the following **except:**
    A. assess the respiratory rate.
    B. listen for air movement.
    C. assess the heart rate.
    D. assess the rise and fall of the chest.

87. Signs of adequate ventilation in an adult include all of the following **except:**
    A. respiratory rate of 16 breaths per minute.
    B. adequate air movement from the nose and mouth.
    C. slight cyanosis to the oral mucosa.
    D. equal and full chest rise and fall.

88. The size of the tongue in an infant when compared proportionately with that of an adult is:
    A. smaller.
    B. larger.
    C. equal in size.
    D. extremely small.

89. What is the narrowest portion of the upper airway for infants and children under 10 years of age?
    A. posterior oral pharynx
    B. the epiglottic opening
    C. glottic opening
    D. the cricoid cartilage

90. You arrive on scene to find a frantic mother screaming that her daughter cannot breathe. The infant is making high-pitched sounds on inspiration, has good color, is alert, and is gasping for air. You suspect what problem?
    A. acute exacerbation of bronchitis
    B. partial airway obstruction
    C. asthma attack
    D. complete airway obstruction

91. Your treatment for an adult patient with a partial airway obstruction as compared with a complete obstruction varies in that:
    A. in a complete obstruction, oxygen is provided by nonrebreather mask, and no oxygen is given in a partial obstruction.
    B. in a partial obstruction, you would attempt to view the obstruction, whereas in a complete obstruction no visualization is performed.
    C. in a partial obstruction, you would instruct the patient to cough, whereas in a complete obstruction you would deliver abdominal thrusts.
    D. in the partial obstruction, priority is placed on removing the obstruction, whereas for a complete obstruction, immediate transport is the key management.

92. Signs indicative of a complete airway obstruction include all of the following **except:**
    A. the patient does not cry or talk.
    B. central and/or core cyanosis may be present.
    C. the patient will cough forcefully.
    D. there is no chest rise or fall.

93. During the mechanical process of inspiration:

   A. the diaphragm contracts along with the intercostal muscles, causing expansion of the thoracic cavity.

   B. the diaphragm contracts, pulling the ribs inward and causing expansion of the chest.

   C. the diaphragm relaxes, allowing the intercostal muscles to contract and thus causing inspiration.

   D. the intercostal muscles contract, causing the ribs to flare out and pull up on the diaphragm.

94. The process of exchange of oxygen and carbon dioxide at the cell is known as:

   A. oxygenation.

   B. ventilation.

   C. inspiration.

   D. respiration.

95. This structure has a common opening for the respiratory tract and the digestive system.

   A. larynx

   B. esophagus

   C. trachea

   D. pharynx

96. A common cause of upper airway obstruction in a young child is flexion of the head. The flexion is commonly caused by:

   A. the child's head being proportionately smaller than the rest of the body.

   B. the trachea being underdeveloped.

   C. the child's tongue being so big it forces the forward flexion.

   D. the head being disproportionately larger, causing flexion of the head.

97. You are called to a residence for a man who is having difficulty breathing. While you are assessing your patient, his wife hands you the telephone stating it's the family doctor. The doctor identifies herself and orders you to administer two puffs of the wife's inhaler because it sounds as if the husband is suffering from the same type of asthma attacks his wife does. You should:

   A. follow the order since it was given by a physician.

   B. advise the physician that you will only follow her orders if she meets you at the emergency room and signs your run report.

   C. explain to the physician that it is against your protocol to help administer the medication since it is not prescribed for your patient.

   D. tell the physician you can perform her order if she writes a prescription for the medication for your patient.

98. Asthma is an example of a(n) _____ airway disease and epiglottitis is a(n) _____ airway disease.

   A. upper, lower

   B. lower, upper

   C. upper, upper

   D. lower, lower

99. A tripod position is a sign of:

   A. severe respiratory distress.

   B. hypoglycemia.

   C. stroke.

   D. heat emergency.

100. The term used to describe a patient in respiratory arrest is:

   A. dyspnea.

   B. bradypnea.

   C. tachypnea.

   D. apnea.

101. Choose the sign or symptom that best indicates severe respiratory distress.
    A. A patient speaks full sentences between breaths.
    B. A patient has a bluish-gray skin color on the neck.
    C. A 10-year-old is breathing 30 times each minute.
    D. A 4-month-old is breathing with abdominal muscles.

102. While assessing a patient who complains of difficulty breathing, you hear stridor when the patient inhales. This is a sign of:
    A. traumatic flail segment.
    B. tension pneumothorax.
    C. sucking chest wound.
    D. partial airway obstruction.

103. All of the following are late signs of respiratory distress in the infant and child **except:**
    A. head bobbing.
    B. slow heart rate.
    C. high blood pressure.
    D. fast breathing rate.

104. You are treating a patient in respiratory distress. You are unsure if the patient needs positive pressure ventilation. You should immediately:
    A. administer oxygen via nonrebreather mask.
    B. provide positive pressure ventilation.
    C. insert a nasopharyngeal airway.
    D. place the patient in the Trendelenburg position.

105. A late sign of respiratory failure in an infant that indicates the need for positive pressure ventilation is:
    A. loss of muscle tone (limp appearance).
    B. cyanosis of the hands and feet.
    C. increased heart rate (tachycardia).
    D. prolonged exhalation and nasal flaring.

106. You are treating an apprehensive child who is experiencing difficulty breathing. The child will not tolerate the nonrebreather mask and continuously removes it from his face. You should:
    A. do nothing because the child cannot be in distress if he can resist treatment.
    B. have a parent hold the mask near the child's face to deliver the oxygen.
    C. speak to the child calmly while holding the mask over his mouth and nose.
    D. place the child on a nasal cannula at 10 lpm and reassure him.

107. You are treating a child who complains of a fever and a sore throat. The child is sitting upright, has his neck jutted out, and is drooling. You should:
    A. inspect inside the child's mouth and oropharynx with a tongue depressor.
    B. perform a finger sweep of the mouth to remove any foreign materials.
    C. provide oxygen by nonrebreather mask and begin immediate transport.
    D. suction the secretions from the oropharynx with the hard suction catheter.

108. You are treating a 4-year-old patient with a sore throat and fever. When the patient coughs, it sounds like a barking seal. You know this as the hallmark sign of:
    A. croup, resulting in swelling of the larynx, trachea, and bronchi.
    B. croup, resulting in constriction of the bronchioles.
    C. epiglottitis, resulting in swelling of the epiglottis in the upper airway.
    D. epiglottitis, resulting in upper airway obstruction from a foreign body.

ALLERGIES AND ANAPHYLAXIS

109. All the following are signs and symptoms of an allergic reaction **except:**

    A. warm, tingling feeling in the face, mouth, feet, and tongue.

    B. decreased heart rate.

    C. tightness in the throat and/or the chest.

    D. urticaria and pruritis.

110. During an allergic reaction, which of the following is an effect (are effects) on the respiratory system?

    A. swelling at the level of the larynx, causing airway compromise

    B. spasms of the bronchi, causing wheezing

    C. significant swelling of the tongue, causing airway compromise

    D. all of the above

111. Your patient was stung by a yellow jacket and now is complaining of difficulty swallowing, shortness of breath, and tightness in the chest. Your primary concern in this patient is to:

    A. provide aggressive airway management with positive ventilation if necessary.

    B. place him or her in a left lateral recumbent position.

    C. activate ALS due to rapid respiratory deterioration.

    D. apply the AED for impending cardiac arrest.

112. Your patient states she is "deathly" allergic to peanuts and she just ate a pie cooked with peanut oil. She appears to be itching all over and has watery eyes and hives on her arms. The patient has no other complaints. You would classify this as a _____ and treat it by _____.

    A. severe reaction, immediately administering epinephrine

    B. mild reaction, positive pressure ventilation

    C. mild reaction, providing reassurance and supplemental oxygen

    D. severe reaction, providing reassurance and supplemental oxygen

113. It is important to treat all possible cases of allergic reactions as serious because:

    A. a mild reaction can rapidly progress to severe anaphylaxis.

    B. infection from the stinger can cause loss of an extremity.

    C. allergic reactions can mimic other more serious medical emergencies.

    D. the patient may develop hives and itching.

114. A sign of anaphylactic shock that would require epinephrine administration is:

    A. hypotension (low blood pressure).

    B. tachycardia (rapid heart rate).

    C. hives.

    D. flushed skin.

115. A sign of anaphylaxis is:

    A. increased systolic blood pressure.

    B. nasal flaring and rapid breathing.

    C. weakness to one side of the body.

    D. all of the above.

116. Your patient took a new medication today and began experiencing difficulty breathing. When you arrive on-scene you hear a high-pitched sound as she breathes. This sound is indicative of:

    A. lower bronchial obstruction.

    B. main stem bronchi obstruction.

    C. laryngeal swelling.

    D. fluid in the alveoli.

117. When managing the patient with an allergic reaction, it is important to constantly reassess the:

    A. flushing of the skin.

    B. hives.

    C. itching.

    D. stridorous respirations.

118. Epinephrine by auto-injector:
    A. is carried on all First Responder units.
    B. is a sublingual injection.
    C. does not require an order to administer it.
    D. is prescribed to the patient.

119. You arrive on the scene and find a patient who states he is allergic to shellfish. He has hives, itching, and slightly flushed skin. His BP is 128/78 mmHg, HR is 102 bpm, and RR is 18/minute. Which of the following treatments would be inappropriate?
    A. epinephrine administration by auto-injector into the thigh
    B. high-flow oxygen by nonrebreather mask set at 15 lpm
    C. positioning the patient in the position most comfortable for him or her
    D. reassess and wait for transport unit to provide treatment while en route to the hospital

120. You suspect your patient is suffering from an anaphylactic reaction, and the airway is compromised by a swollen larynx. The most effective method of managing this obstruction is:
    A. providing positive pressure ventilation.
    B. positioning the patient's head.
    C. inserting an oropharyngeal airway.
    D. suctioning the upper airway often.

121. Which of the following is the correct administration procedure for a prescribed epinephrine auto-injector?
    A. Push the auto-injector firmly against the patient's upper hip between the thigh and the lower back; hold in place for 1 second.
    B. Push the auto-injector firmly against the patient's upper arm between the elbow and the shoulder; hold in place until half the vial is delivered.
    C. Push the auto-injector firmly against the patient's thigh midway between the waist and the knee; hold in place until all the medication is delivered.
    D. Push the auto-injector firmly against the patient's lower leg midway between the knee and the ankle; hold in place until all the medication is delivered.

122. You have administered epinephrine to an anaphylactic patient. She complains of a headache, dizziness, chest pain, and increased heart rate. These signs are indicative of:
    A. incorrect administration.
    B. overdose of epinephrine.
    C. side effects of epinephrine.
    D. allergic reaction to the drug.

123. Which of the following is a contraindication of epinephrine administration in anaphylaxis?
    A. There are no contraindications in anaphylaxis.
    B. elderly patient
    C. infants and children
    D. stridorous respiration

SCENARIO

Questions 124–126 refer to the following scenario:

You and your partner Ashley are restocking the First Response unit after a serious automobile accident on I–95. The station alerting system sounds, "Unit one respond to an allergic reaction at 1729 17th Avenue. Time out 13:52." As you approach the scene, you are met at the street by a frantic husband who states, "It's my wife; she was stung by a bee and now she can't breathe." You and Ashley enter the house and find a 36-year-old female sitting on a kitchen chair. She is in a tripod position and looks at you and Ashley with fright-filled eyes. She is breathing approximately 40 times a minute. Ashley states she can hear audible wheezes; the skin is flushed and dry with urticaria (hives) covering the chest and back. The patient begins to slump over in the chair. Her pulse rate is 134 bpm.

124. From the information provided, select the most appropriate immediate treatment for this patient.
    A. Place a constricting band above injection site.
    B. Immediately wash the injection site.
    C. Provide positive pressure ventilation.
    D. Administer oxygen by nonrebreather mask.

125. The patient's husband locates and gives you the patient's epinephrine auto-injector. You should do which of the following next?
    A. Obtain an order from medical direction to administer the patient's prescribed epinephrine by auto-injector.
    B. In this situation, there is no need to administer the epinephrine auto-injector.
    C. This patient is not having an anaphylactic reaction and should not receive epinephrine by auto-injector.
    D. Administer epinephrine by auto-injector after you have applied constricting bands below the injection site.

126. After you have administered epinephrine by auto-injector, the patient becomes very pale and the heart rate increases to 150 bpm. The patient becomes very anxious and states she feels as if she is going to vomit. The signs and symptoms indicate:
    A. an epinephrine overdose.
    B. a common side effect of epinephrine.
    C. the patient's condition is worsening.
    D. incorrect administration of epinephrine.

TRAUMA EMERGENCIES 5-2 AND 5-3

127. Your patient has a laceration to the leg; the wound is bleeding heavily in a steady flow that is dark red. You suspect the patient is bleeding from a:
    A. capillary.
    B. artery.
    C. arteriole.
    D. vein.

128. Which of the following best describes arterial bleeding?
    A. dark red and flows steadily from wounds
    B. bright red, under high pressure, and typically spurts
    C. oozing flow that usually clots spontaneously
    D. steady flow that is easily controlled due to pressure

129. Your adult patient has lost a large amount of blood from a suspected abdominal injury and internal bleeding. The patient is in shock. He is breathing 24 times a minute with good rise and fall of the chest. You should manage the patient by:
    A. administering fluids by mouth to replace the lost blood volume.
    B. continuing with treatment based on the assessment findings.
    C. administering positive pressure ventilation by pocket mask.
    D. giving epinephrine by auto-injector.

130. Your patient is bleeding from a laceration to the forearm. The artery or pressure point that should be utilized to control bleeding is the:
    A. ulna artery.
    B. radial artery.
    C. femoral artery.
    D. brachial artery.

131. A tourniquet should be:
    A. made of a narrow, flat material.
    B. covered with a bandage.
    C. used when direct pressure and pressure points fail.
    D. applied directly over a joint and tight enough to eliminate distal pulses.

132. If bleeding from the lower leg is not controlled with direct pressure, you should also:
    A. utilize a pressure point.
    B. elevate the extremity.
    C. use a tourniquet.
    D. rapidly apply an air splint.

133. Internal bleeding from blunt trauma:
    A. is usually very obvious to identify.
    B. should be suspected with unexplained shock.
    C. never results in severe blood loss.
    D. can be ruled out if the abdomen is rigid.

134. Your patient presents with signs of severe hypoperfusion after falling from a tree. You do not find any signs of external bleeding. Your partner is providing manual in-line spinal stabilization, and you have applied a nonrebreather mask at 15 lpm. Your best immediate action for this patient is to:
    A. do a detailed physical exam until you find the exact injury site.
    B. assist the EMS crew to prepare the patient for immediate transport to the hospital.
    C. delay transport until all of the injuries are dressed and bandaged.
    D. only provide treatment if the heart rate is elevated.

135. Which of the following early signs would alert you that your 20-year-old patient may have internal bleeding?
    A. decreased blood pressure
    B. deep slow breathing
    C. capillary refill that is less than 2 seconds
    D. thready pulse rate of 110 bpm

136. Which of the following is **not** a sign or symptom associated with blood loss and shock?
    A. nausea and vomiting
    B. restlessness
    C. hot, dry skin
    D. marked thirst

137. The outermost layer of the skin is known as the:
    A. epidermis.
    B. endodermis.
    C. dermis.
    D. subcutaneous layer.

138. You are preparing to treat a patient with a soft-tissue injury. Which action should be taken first?
    A. airway control and ventilation management
    B. oxygen administration
    C. body substance isolation precautions
    D. bleeding control

139. A type of soft-tissue injury that is caused by scraping, rubbing, or shearing away of the epidermis is called a(n):
    A. abrasion.
    B. puncture.
    C. avulsion.
    D. laceration.

140. Which type of dressing should be used to treat an open chest wound?
    A. water-soaked gauze
    B. plastic wrap
    C. 4 × 4 sterile dressing
    D. large abdominal pad

141. Your patient has an open chest wound; the best method to secure the occlusive dressing should be:
    A. taping one side.
    B. taping two sides.
    C. taping three sides.
    D. taping all four sides.

142. The treatment for an open abdominal wound with an evisceration should include:
    A. replacing the abdominal organs.
    B. using an absorbent dressing.
    C. keeping the patient's leg flat.
    D. covering the dressing with a bulky material.

143. Your patient has been burned by a grease fire. Large blisters have formed on the surface of the skin. This is a:
    A. superficial burn.
    B. full thickness burn.
    C. partial thickness burn.
    D. first-degree burn.

144. Your patient is suffering intense pain from a scald burn. The burn includes the epidermis, as well as portions of the dermis. This burn is classified as a:
    A. partial thickness burn.
    B. superficial burn.
    C. full thickness burn.
    D. partial eschar burn.

145. A partial thickness burn involves:
    A. the epidermis only.
    B. the epidermis and dermis.
    C. the dermis and muscle.
    D. the dermis, fat, and muscle.

146. A full thickness burn may appear:
    A. dry, hard, and leathery.
    B. slightly red with blisters.
    C. pink to red.
    D. red with blisters.

147. The most critical type of burn is a:
    A. first-degree burn.
    B. full thickness burn.
    C. partial thickness burn.
    D. second degree burn.

148. In managing a burn, special emphasis should be placed upon:
    A. preventing further contamination and injury.
    B. removing clothing that has adhered to the area.
    C. leaving jewelry in the burned areas in place.
    D. calculation of the exact body surface area involved.

149. Which of the following is **inappropriate** treatment for the patient suffering from a full thickness burn?
    A. Cover the entire burn area with a dry sterile dressing.
    B. Apply a sterile antiseptic burn ointment on the burn.

C. Douse smoldering clothing with water.
    D. Conserve heat loss by covering the patient.

150. Which of the following statements is **incorrect** pertaining to the application of pressure dressings?
    A. If blood soaks through, leave the dressing in place and apply more dressings.
    B. Air splints can be used to apply pressure and hold dressings in place on the extremities.
    C. Loss of a distal pulse indicates the dressing is too tight.
    D. The wound should be covered with several bulky dressings.

151. Which of the following impaled objects may be removed in the prehospital setting?
    A. screwdriver embedded in the chest
    B. pitchfork impaled through the foot
    C. pencil impaled through the cheek
    D. knife embedded in the upper leg

152. When managing an electrical burn, you should:
    A. immediately apply the AED in case the patient goes into cardiac arrest.
    B. check for both a source and ground burn injury.
    C. apply burn ointment to any areas that have been burned.
    D. apply oxygen only if the pateint complains of shortness of breath.

153. Your patient has suffered an electrical burn. Which of the following statements is **incorrect?**
    A. Patients with electrical burns may be treated with the AED and CPR.
    B. Treatment for a source wound is the same as for other thermal burns.
    C. Injury is usually limited to the area around the source and ground wounds.
    D. Patients with burns that appear insignificant are treated as critical injuries.

154. You are treating a patient with a painful, swollen and deformed upper arm. You suspect which bone is injured?
    A. scapula
    B. radius
    C. ulna
    D. humerus

155. A general rule for splinting is to:
    A. check the pulse, motor function, and sensation before splinting.
    B. check the pulse and sensation before and after splinting.
    C. check the pulse, motor function, and sensation after splinting.
    D. check the pulse, motor function, and sensation before and after splinting.

156. Your patient was struck by a car while riding his bicycle. He complains of pain in his right upper arm and lower back. Which of the following treatments should **not** be performed after splinting the arm?
    A. elevate the extremity
    B. dress any open wounds
    C. apply cold packs
    D. assess motor function

157. Your patient has fallen while skating and complains of pain and swelling to the elbow. You should immobilize the:
    A. joint above the elbow joint only.
    B. joint above and below the elbow.
    C. bone above the elbow joint only.
    D. bones above and below the elbow.

158. Your patient has an obviously deformed, painful, and swollen injury to the tibia. The foot is cyanotic and lacks a pulse. The best immediate action for you to take is to:
    A. transport immediately without applying a splint, and support the leg manually.
    B. apply the splint to the leg in the position found and transport immediately.

    C. make one attempt to align the extremity by applying gentle manual traction.
    D. make up to three attempts to align the extremity by applying firm traction.

159. Which statement is **false** pertaining to splinting a painful, swollen, or deformed extremity?
    A. Motor, sensory, and distal pulses are assessed both prior to and after splinting.
    B. Both the above and below joints are immobilized when a long bone is injured.
    C. Traction is applied to protruding bones until the bones retract below the skin.
    D. Do not attempt to realign a deformed knee injury.

160. The nervous system that consists of the brain and spinal cord is known as the:
    A. peripheral nervous system.
    B. central nervous system.
    C. voluntary nervous system.
    D. autonomic nervous system.

161. The portion of the skeletal system that protects the brain is the:
    A. vertebrae.
    B. cranium.
    C. basilar skull.
    D. ischium.

162. Which of the following signs or symptoms of spinal injury is rarely seen?
    A. numbness, weakness, or tingling in the arms
    B. pain without movement
    C. obvious deformity of the spine
    D. paralysis of the extremities

163. When performing the initial assessment on a patient with a suspected spine injury, you will open and maintain the airway by:
    A. performing the cervical traction maneuver.
    B. performing the lateral lift maneuver.
    C. performing the head-tilt, chin-lift maneuver.
    D. performing the jaw-thrust maneuver.

164. Placing a patient with a spinal injury on a long spine board is ideally performed by how many rescuers?
    A. two
    B. three
    C. four
    D. five

165. To determine the proper size of a rigid cervical spine immobilization collar, measure the distance from the top of the shoulder to the:
    A. level of the larynx.
    B. bottom of the jaw line.
    C. level of C-7.
    D. bottom of the earlobe.

166. You arrive on the scene of an automobile crash and find your patient walking around the scene. The patient complains of neck pain. The correct way to immobilize this patient to minimize movement of the spine is to:
    A. use the standing long board technique to take the patient down.
    B. have the patient sit down on the long board.
    C. use the logrolling technique with a long board.
    D. place the short spinal device on the standing patient.

167. A vest-type immobilization device or a short spine board is used to immobilize a:
    A. standing patient.
    B. supine patient.
    C. seated patient.
    D. rapid-extrication patient.

168. Your patient has been critically injured in a vehicle crash. The patient's injuries are severe, and he must be transported immediately. You should extricate the patient, using the:
    A. short spinal extrication device.
    B. rapid extrication technique.
    C. corset-type immobilization device.
    D. standing long board technique.

169. Rapid extrication is indicated in all of the following patient situations **except:**
    A. an unsafe scene.
    B. a stable patient.
    C. a patient blocking access to a critical patient.
    D. an unstable patient.

170. Which of the following cases would require you to remove a helmet?
    A. The patient has an altered mental status.
    B. The patient complains of head pain.
    C. The patient is in cardiac arrest.
    D. The patient complains of neck pain.

171. The two basic types of helmets are the:
    A. sports and motorcycle.
    B. OSHA and sports.
    C. construction and sports.
    D. construction and motorcycle.

172. When you are dealing with an injured football player with a cervical spine injury:
    A. the helmet should never be removed under any circumstances.
    B. the helmet should be left in place unless a critical need requires removal.
    C. the helmet should only be removed by using a special cutting tool.
    D. the helmet should always be removed.

SCENARIO

Questions 173–175 refer to the following scenario:

It is just after 12 A.M. on a Friday night. You have responded to a motor vehicle accident. The patient is in her mid-20s and is walking about the scene. The patient's car struck a tree, and significant damage is noted to the front of the car. The patient appears distraught as you approach. Her right eye is swollen shut and she has a laceration over the left eye. She tells you she had "too much to drink." She is concerned about her car. She complains of neck pain.

173. Given this situation you should:
    A. have the patient walk to the First Response vehicle and initiate spinal immobilization.
    B. have the patient lie down on the ground and initiate spinal immobilization.
    C. secure the patient's cervical spine and initiate a standing takedown.
    D. have the patient sit down and initiate seated spinal immobilization techniques.

174. The patient suddenly begins to complain of a severe headache and dizziness. You should:
    A. immediately repeat your initial assessment.
    B. insert an orophyarngeal airway and begin ventilation.
    C. contact medical control and ask for assistance.
    D. perform a head-tilt chin-lift manuever to open the airway.

175. Her level of consciousness continues to decline, and she now only responds to deep, painful stimuli. You note snoring respirations. You should:
    A. begin positive pressure ventilation at 24 breaths per minute.
    B. reposition the jaw and insert an oropharyngeal airway.

    C. wait for the EMS crew arrival before providing any additional treatment.
    D. give the patient a glucose solution and place her on her left side.

SCENARIO

Questions 176–178 refer to the following scenario:

You and your partner Bill are responding to a burn emergency. Upon arrival you find a 52-year-old patient lying supine on the ground next to a gas grill. Bill makes patient contact and finds the patient awake and responsive with an adequate airway. The patient states he was cleaning his grill with gasoline when it exploded and burned him.

176. The patient has sustained burns that encircle both arms. The burns appear dark brown, leathery and charred. You classify this burn as a:
    A. superficial thickness burn.
    B. half thickness burn.
    C. partial thickness burn.
    D. full thickness burn.

177. Which of the following would cause you to categorize the patient as having a critical burn?
    A. burn involving a volatile substance
    B. patient's age
    C. possibility of breathing in a toxic chemical
    D. circumferential burns to the upper extremities

178. You should treat the burns by:
    A. covering the burns with a dry sterile dressing.
    B. applying a burn ointment because the burns are circumferential.
    C. breaking any blisters and removing the charred skin.
    D. applying ice to the burn area for at least 30 minutes.

SCENARIO

Questions 179–181 refer to the following scenario:

You arrive on the scene and find a male patient in his mid-20s who fell from a rocky ledge about 50 feet. Once you gain access to the patient, you find he responds to painful stimuli with flexion of his extremities while arching his back. He is bleeding from his mouth, ears, and nose. His respirations are 35/minute and shallow. His radial pulse is present and bounding.

179. Your first immediate action is to:

A. suction the mouth and apply a nonrebreather mask at 15 lpm if available.

B. move the patient up the embankment.

C. cut away the clothing to inspect for other injuries.

D. suction the airway, insert an oropharyngeal airway, and begin ventilation.

180. Which of the signs provides the strongest indication that the patient is suffering from a head injury?

A. the blood coming from the nose, ears, and mouth

B. a respiratory rate of 35/minute

C. flexion of the extremities and arching of the back with painful stimuli

D. strong radial pulses

181. The best treatment you could provide this patient is to:

A. administer oral glucose to allow the brain cells to function.

B. maintain a patent airway and continue to provide effective ventilation.

C. place the patient in a semi-seated position to decrease pressure to the head.

D. place the patient in a lateral recumbent position to allow the blood to drain.

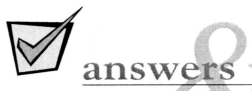

answers & rationales

Following each rationale, you will find a reference to the corresponding D.O.T. objective. A rationale marked with an asterisk denotes material supplemental to the First Responder curriculum. Also included after each rationale are references to where the question topic may be covered in Brady First Responder textbooks. **"FR7" refers to** *First Responder, 7e* (Bergeron, Bizjak, Krause, Le Baudour). **"FRASA" refers to** *First Responder: A Skills Approach,* **7e** (Limmer, Karren, Hafen).

ALTERED MENTAL STATUS AND DIABETIC EMERGENCIES

1.

C. Micronase is an oral hypoglycemia agent. This patient is exhibiting signs of a low blood sugar level (hypoglycemia). (5-1.1) (FR7 p. 250; FRASA pp. 270–271)

2.

D. A patient suffering from low blood sugar level (hypoglycemia) will exhibit a rapid onset of signs and symptoms to include an altered mental status due to the glucose deficiency; tachycardia; and pale, cool, clammy skin. (5-1.1) (FR7 p. 250; FRASA pp. 270–271)

3.

A. A patient must have an intact gag reflex and the ability to swallow in order to receive instant oral glucose. (5-1.2) (FR7 p. 250; FRASA pp. 271–272)

4.

C. The entire tube of glucose should be placed on a tongue depressor and placed between the gum and the cheek to dissolve in the patient's mouth. Rubbing the area may increase the absorption rate. (5-1.4) (FR7 p. 560; FRASA p. 272)

5.

D. Due to the decreased level of consciousness and snoring respirations, this patient should receive nothing by mouth. The treatment would be to open the airway, insert an adjunct airway, and continue the assessment. (5-1.4) (FR7 p. 250; FRASA p. 269)

6.

A. The patient who is unable to protect his or her own airway should not receive oral glucose. (5-1.4) (FR7 p. 250; FRASA pp. 271–272)

7.

D. The treatment for this patient is to maintain an open airway, administer high-flow oxygen if available and able to do so according to your protocol, suction if necessary, assist ventilation if necessary, position the patient on his side, and transport. Do not administer oral glucose or any other glucose solution by mouth due to the altered mental status and the risk of aspiration. Three criteria must be met before administering oral glucose: 1) the patient must have an altered mental status, 2) the patient must have a history of diabetes controlled by medication, and 3) the patient must be alert enough to swallow. This patient only responded to tactile stimulation and would not be able to protect his own airway. (5-1.4) (FR7 p. 250; FRASA p. 269)

8.

A. If the patient becomes unresponsive while you are administering oral glucose, remove the tongue depressor and reassess the airway, breathing, and circulation. Placing the unresponsive patient in a semi-sitting position may compromise the airway. Do not try to remove the glucose from the patient's cheek. This is a small amount and will not likely compromise the airway. Do not administer additional glucose to the unresponsive patient. (5-1.4) (FR7 p. 560; FRASA pp. 269–271)

9.

B. Airway maintenance is the priority of care in the patient suffering from an altered mental status. (FR7 p. 244; FRASA p. 268)

10.

D. Airway management is the priority in patient care, followed by positioning. (5-1.2) (FR7 p. 101; FRASA p. 269)

96

11.

C. A patient with an altered mental status who has no evidence of trauma to the spine should be positioned in a left lateral recumbent position. Even though you are not sure whether the patient can understand what you are saying, it is important for you to continuously explain to the patient what you are doing. Some patients with an altered mental status can hear and understand you even though they present with an altered mental state. (5-1.4) (FR7 pp. 148–149; FRASA pp. 269)

ALTERED MENTAL STATUS—STROKE

12.

D. Aphasia is the inability to speak. Hemiplegia is paralysis to one side of the body. Hemiparesis is weakness to one side of the body. All are signs of a stroke. (5-1.3) (FR7 p. 244; FRASA p. 272)

13.

C. A TIA is a transient ischemic attack. TIAs are often called "mini strokes." They differ in that the effects are only temporary and do not cause any permanent neurological dysfunction. The signs and symptoms of a TIA resolve within 24 hours and leave no permanent cognitive, temporary, or motor deficits. (5-1.3) (FRASA p. 272)

14.

B. One of the most common findings associated with a hemorrhagic stroke is a sudden onset of "the worst headache" the patient has suffered. Hemorrhagic strokes are commonly associated with high blood pressure (hypertension). The severe headache is caused by the increased intracranial pressure associated with rupture of an artery and collection of blood in the skull. (1-5.3) (FR7 p. 244; FRASA p. 274)

15.

D. A stiff neck is a late sign of stroke caused by hemorrhage. Seizures, headache, and unequal pupils often occur early in a stroke. (5-1.3) (FR7 pp. 244–245)

16.

C. Severe intermittent abdominal pain is not a sign or symptom of stroke. Hemiplegia is the medical term used to describe one-sided paralysis. Loss of bowel and bladder control and unequal pupils or vision disturbances are common signs and symptoms associated with a stroke. (5-1.3) (FR7 pp. 244–245; FRASA p. 272–274)

17.

B. This patient has signs and symptoms of a stroke. This patient awoke with these symptoms, which should cause you to suspect a medical problem rather than a traumatic injury. Hypoglycemia (low blood sugar level) may present with all of the signs and symptoms except unequal pupils. (5-1.3) (FR7 pp. 244–245; FRASA p. 274)

POISONING/OVERDOSE

18.

B. Unequal pupils may indicate a brain injury from a stroke or trauma. Patients with poisoning or an overdose may have dilated or constricted pupils; however, the pupils remain equal. (5-1.3) (FR7 p. 255; FRASA pp. 278–281)

19.

D. Many patients who have overdosed on medications or are poisoned cannot maintain their airway. Your first concern is to open and maintain the patient's airway. Manual airway maneuvers and the use of airway adjuncts like the nasopharyngeal airway or the oropharyngeal airway may be necessary to maintain an open airway. (5-1.4) (FR7 p. 256; FRASA p. 320)

20.

B. You must immediately provide positive pressure ventilation to any patient with respirations that become inadequate. (5-1.4) (FR7 pp. 256–257; FRASA pp. 319–320)

21.

C. A patient who has overdosed on blood pressure medication is a good candidate for activated charcoal. Activated charcoal can be used up to 4 hours after ingestion of some medications. Activated charcoal is contraindicated in liquid bleach and ammonia. Activated charcoal is an adsorbent that is used in ingested poisonings, not inhalation. (5-1.4) (FR7 pp. 560–561; FRASA p. 280)

22.

C. Activated charcoal is very porous; thus, it adsorbs the poison and inhibits the absorption into the body. Some poisons have slow absorption rates that allow activated charcoal to be used up to 4 hours after ingestion. (5-1.4) (FR7 pp. 560–561; FRASA p. 280)

23.

D. The routes of entry into the human body include ingestion, inhalation, injection, and absorption. (5-1.3) (FR7 p. 253; FRASA p. 278)

24.

C. The medication is absorbed under the tongue in the very vascular oral mucosa. (5-1.3) (FR7 p. 253; FRASA p. 281)

25.

B. An injection is the mode of entry of a substance through a break in the skin. The break can be caused by a stinger, needle, or being bitten. (5-1.3) (FR7 p. 253; FRASA p. 281–282)

26.

C. Dry powders should be brushed off before the area is irrigated. Many chemicals are inactive in the powder form, but are activated, or become more activated, when they come into contact with water, creating a reaction that may create heat and cause further burning. (5-1.4) (FR7 p. 259; FRASA p. 281)

27.

D. The first priority for the First Responder is always scene safety. The scene in this case is obviously unsafe because of the chlorine leak. The scene must be managed by personnel trained in hazardous material who have the appropriate equipment to extricate the patients. (5-1.4) (FR7 p. 257; FRASA p. 281, 549)

28.

B. The patient should be placed in the lateral recumbent position, also known as the coma or recovery position, to prevent aspiration of secretions, vomitus, blood, and other substances. (5-1.2) (FR7 p. 247; FRASA p. 276)

29.

C. Whenever you have a question concerning an overdose or poisoning, you should contact the poison control center. It provides the most updated information. (5-1.4) (FR7 p. 253; FRASA p. 279)

30.

B. Treatment of this patient includes maintaining a patent airway, insertion of a nasopharyngeal airway, and providing positive pressure ventilation. You should never give anything by mouth to a patient who has an altered level of consciousness who cannot protect his own airway. This could lead to aspiration of the substance. (5-1.4) (FR7 pp. 256–257; FRASA pp. 279–280)

31.

A. Activated charcoal is only useful for poisonings that occur by ingestion. (5-1.4) (FR7 p. 256, 560; FRASA p. 280)

32.

C. The contraindications for the use of activated charcoal include the patient who has an altered mental status, has swallowed acids or alkalis (hydrochloric acid, bleach, ammonia, ethanol), or is unable to swallow. (5-1.4) (FR7 pp. 560–561; FRASA p. 280)

33.

C. It is important to determine if the patient is suffering from a medical condition or the effects of drugs and/or alcohol. Many medical conditions can mimic the effect of drugs and alcohol. Search the area immediately around the patient for evidence of drug or alcohol use. (5-1.3) (FR7 pp. 274–275; FRASA p. 318)

34.

A. Phencyclidine is also known as PCP. PCP patients may become agitated and enraged if this technique is utilized. The "Talk Down Technique" includes making the patient feel welcome, identifying yourself clearly, reassuring the patient, helping the patient verbalize what is taking place, repeating simple concrete statements, and forewarning the patient of actions to be taken. (5-1.4) (FR7 p. 271, 276; FRASA p. 313)

SEIZURES

35.

B. A seizure is a sudden and temporary alteration caused by the electrical discharge from active foci in the brain. (5-1.5) (FR7 p. 246; FRASA p. 275)

36.

D. The sequence of events starts with the aura, next the tonic phase lasting 15–20 seconds, then the clonic (tonic-clonic) phase lasting 30 seconds to 5 minutes, and finally the postictal phase, which lasts from 5–30 minutes. (5-1.5) (FRASA pp. 275–276)

37.

D. All the conditions can cause irritation to the neurons of the brain, which can trigger a seizure. (5-1.5) (FR7 p. 246; FRASA p. 274)

38.

C. Treatment for an actively seizing patient is supportive. Always protect the patient from harm, monitor the airway, suction if necessary. Apply oxygen if you are able to do so, and assist ventilation if necessary. Never pry or force anything into the patient's mouth. This can cause further damage. (5-1.6) (FR7 p. 247; FRASA p. 276)

39.

C. Status epilepticus is a dire medical emergency. These patients need immediate medical intervention. (5-1.5) (FRASA p. 276)

40.

A. The nasopharyngeal airway can be inserted in an actively seizing patient to provide a means of airway control without harming the patient. (5-1.6) (FR7 p. 128; FRASA p. 124)

41.

C. This condition is status epilepticus. This is a dire medical emergency that requires aggressive airway control and positive pressure ventilation with supplemental oxygen. The patient should be transported rapidly. (5-1.5) (FRASA p. 276)

42.

C. The aura is a warning that a seizure is about to occur. This stage can present as a sound, twitch, or odor; some patients even experience an unusual taste that precedes the seizure. Some patients experience auras; however, many seizure patients do not. (5-1.5) (FRASA p. 275)

43.

A. The postictal phase is known as the recovery phase. During this phase the patient's mental status may range from complete unresponsiveness to confusion. The patient's mental status improves with time. These patients appear exhausted. (5-1.5) (FRASA p. 276)

44.

C. Syncope is commonly known as fainting. Syncope usually occurs when the patient is standing or the patient stands up from a sitting position. Syncope is caused by a lack of blood flow to the brain. This causes the brain to become deprived of oxygen, rendering the patient unconscious for a brief period. This brief period of unconsciousness is usually corrected once the patient falls to a horizontal position. (5-1.5)

45.

B. The best position to place a patient who has experienced a syncopal episode is supine with the legs elevated. A supine position will allow more blood to flow to the brain, increasing cerebral oxygenation. The supine position will also allow you to visually inspect the airway and provide oxygen therapy. (5-1.6) (FR7 p. 314)

46.

B. This emergency situation is most likely a syncopal episode. A syncopal episode usually occurs when the patient is in a standing position and usually resolves after the patient is placed in a horizontal position. The skin is usually moist and pale. This also improves when the patient is lying on the floor. (5-1.5)

47.

D. A febrile seizure that lasts longer than 15 minutes would be considered significant. This patient would require aggressive management. (5-1.5) (FR7 p. 475; FRASA p. 512)

ENVIRONMENTAL—HEAT AND COLD EMERGENCIES

48.

D. The majority of heat lost through the human body is from the head, feet, and hands through radiation. (5-1.7) (FRASA p. 289)

49.

C. Water conducts heat away from the human body 240 times faster than any other mechanism. (5-1.7) (FRASA p. 289)

50.

B. Signs of early hypothermia include shivering, muscle cramps, and rapid heart rate. Bradycardia (slow heart rate) occurs later in hypothermia with more severe decreases in body core temperature. (5-1.7) (FR7 p. 267; FRASA pp. 291–292)

51.

A. The core body temperature will drop 25–30 times faster because the body is in contact with cold water molecules. The body's temperature will cool to that of the temperature of the ambient environment around it, in this case, the water temperature. (5-1.7) (FRASA p. 289)

52.

D. All the answers are true of the elderly, which places them at a greater risk for heat emergencies. (5-1.9) (FRASA p. 294)

53.

D. This patient is presenting with signs showing that the body's compensatory mechanisms have shut down. This patient can be classified as having heat stroke. The patient needs rapid cooling to prevent cellular breakdown due to the increased body temperature. (5-1.10) (FR7 p. 264; FRASA p. 296)

54.

D. Children suffer from environmental emergencies because of their proportionately larger body surface areas, body fat storages, and the inability to dress for the climate. (5-1.7) (FRASA p. 290)

55.

B. The hypothermic patient should be handled very gently to prevent ventricular fibrillation, which may be caused by rough handling. Don't rub or massage the patient's arms or legs. This may force cold venous blood into the heart, resulting in cardiac arrest. If ventilation is required, avoid hyperventilation; this may cause further cardiac compromise and cool the patient faster if in a cold environment. Defibrillate and provide CPR as needed if the patient is in cardiac arrest. A cold heart does not respond well to defibrillation. (5-1.8) (FR7 p. 267; FRASA p. 292)

56.

C. If you are unable to obtain a pulse and there are no respirations, but patient movement is detected, delay CPR and the use of the AED. Pulses are very difficult to find in hypothermic patients. You should immediately begin positive pressure ventilation. (5-1.8) (FR7 p. 267; FRASA p. 292)

57.

B. Instruct the patient to remain as calm and immobile as possible with just enough effort to remain afloat. Lift the patient from the water in a horizontal or supine position. Remove the wet clothing as quickly and gently as possible to prevent further heat loss and ventricular fibrillation. (5-1.8) (FRASA p. 276)

58.

B. Correct management includes the removal of jewelry. Avoid massaging the affected area and the application of salves or ointments. Blisters that are present should be left intact and should not be broken. (5-1.8) (FR7 p. 269; FRASA p. 293)

59.

D. Rewarming of localized frozen tissue should generally be avoided unless you have a long delay to transport. If performed, use water at 100–110°F. Never use dry heat because it is too difficult to control the temperature. Rewarming of tissue is very painful, and medical control will commonly want the patient to have an analgesic. (5-1.8) (FR7 pp. 268–269; FRASA p. 293)

60.

D. Begin cooling the patient by moving the patient into the shade, in an air-conditioned building or vehicle. This would be followed by removal of clothing; oxygen administration; and rapid cooling with water, cold packs, or other cooling techniques. (5-1.10) (FR7 p. 264; FRASA p. 296)

61.

A. This patient is considered a high priority. Cooling should be continued until the EMS crew arrives on the scene and en route to the hospital. Maintain an airway and monitor the respirations closely. Provide positive pressure ventilation if necessary. (5-1.10) (FR7 p. 263; FRASA p. 295)

62.

D. The patient is suffering from a heat emergency. This is most likely to occur when the temperature is higher than 90°F with a relative humidity of greater than 75 percent. (5-1.9) (FRASA p. 295)

63.

B. Family history is not a predisposing factor that increases the risk of hypothermia (cold emergency). A person's age is a major factor in the risk of hypothermia. The young and old are more likely to suffer from hypothermia. Medical conditions such as head injury, spinal cord injury, stroke, diabetes, and a heart condition can increase the likelihood of hypothermia. Alcohol dilates blood vessels and interferes with the normal thermal regulator mechanisms, which can increase the patient's risk of hypothermia. (5-1.7) (FR7 p. 266; FRASA p. 290)

64.

C. Shivering and goose bumps are the body's first reactions to a decrease in body temperature found in the first stage of hypothermia. The second stage of hypothermia involves a decrease in fine, and then gross, motor function. The fine motor function may be as subtle as a patient's inability to follow simple commands. As the hypothermia continues, the patient may not be able to move the arms or legs. A decrease in the heart rate and respirations is the fourth stage of hypothermia. (5-1.7) (FR7 p. 267; FRASA p. 291)

65.

B. This patient should be placed in a supine (lying flat) position with the feet elevated approximately 8–12 inches. This will increase the blood flow to the brain. If the patient is responsive and not nauseated, administer a half glass of water every 15 minutes. (5-1.8) (FR7 p. 264; FRASA p. 296)

BEHAVIORAL AND PSYCHOLOGICAL CRISIS

66.

B. A person's personality is just one aspect of his or her behavior. Depression and anxiety are classifications of behaviors. (5-1.11) (FR7 p. 270; FRASA p. 312)

67.

C. Society has classified acceptable or "normal" behavior for many situations. Any deviation outside of the norms may be considered abnormal. (5-1.11) (FR7 p. 270; FRASA p. 312)

68.

D. There are many different etiologies including oxygen deficits, altered glucose levels, and other deficiencies that could lead to abnormal behavior. Be sure to assess the patient carefully and check for an organic cause for the behavior. (5-1.11) (FR7 p. 270; FRASA p. 312)

69.

D. Patients who want to hurt themselves often use extreme measures to do so. Others may place themselves in high-risk situations. Report this information to the EMS crew. (5-1.13) (FRASA p. 313)

70.

C. A leading cause of suicide is depression over the loss of a loved one. (5-1.13) (FRASA p. 524)

71.

B. Approximately 80 percent of patients who commit suicide have made a previous attempt. This is one reason why all patients who have suicidal tendencies should be transported. (5-1.13)

72.

C. You should be concerned that the patient may have attempted suicide. You should directly ask the patient if he or she was attempting to kill himself or herself. (5-1.13)

73.

B. Patients who have constructed a plan on how to kill themselves are much more likely to carry out their intentions than those who have no plan. (5-1.13)

74.

B. When a patient informs you that he or she has thought of harming himself or herself and has formulated a plan, you should become highly concerned for your safety and that of the patient's, especially when a gun is involved in the plan. Re-assess the scene safety and retreat if necessary. (5-1.14)

75.

C. Whenever any scene becomes unsafe you should immediately remove yourself from it. Contact law enforcement to handle the weapon. Once the scene is secure, enter it to manage the patient. (5-1.12) (FR7 p. 272; FRASA p. 315)

76.

B. Patients over the age of 40 are more likely to commit suicide. The elderly commonly suffer severe depression and are very likely to commit suicide. Depression in an elderly patient is actually considered a serious emergency. (5-1.13) (FRASA p. 524)

77.

D. When assessing this type of patient, have adequate personnel to help restrain the patient, if necessary. Make sure the scene is free from potential weapons and always have available exit routes. (5-1.14) (FR7 p. 271; FRASA pp. 314–315)

78.

D. All of the factors can cause aggression. Be sure not to rule out an organic cause of aggression. (5-1.11) (FR7 p. 270; FRASA p. 313)

79.

B. Your job is not to be judgmental but rather impartial. You should ask about the patient's intention of killing himself or herself. (5-1.14) (FRASA p. 315)

80.

B. Once a patient is restrained, the restraints should be left on. The patient may be calm one minute and revert back to the aggressive behavior the next. (5-1.14) (FRASA p. 316)

ENRICHMENT

Respiratory

81.

C. The respiratory system includes the larynx, the trachea, and the lungs. The esophagus is part of the gastrointestinal system. (*) (FR7 pp. 99–100; FRASA p. 95)

82.

D. Functions of the nose include warming, filtering, and humidifying inspired air. (*) (FR7 p. 99; FRASA p. 95)

83.

B. The epiglottis is a flap of cartilage that acts like a valve directing air into the trachea and food into the esophagus. (*) (FR7 p. 100; FRASA p. 95)

84.

C. The major muscle of respiration is the diaphragm. It accounts for 60 percent of the respiratory effort. (*) (FR7 p. 98; FRASA p. 96)

85.

B. Early signs of hypoxia are tachycardia (increased heart rate); pale, cool, clammy skin; and tachypnea (increased respiratory rate). (*)

86.

C. To determine the tidal volume, the First Responder must assess the chest rise and fall, listen for sounds of air movement, and determine the respiratory rate. By determining the tidal volume, the First Responder can determine if the patient is breathing adequately. (*) (FR7 p. 100; FRASA pp. 102–103)

87.

C. Cyanosis to the oral mucosa indicates inadequate oxygenation. A respiratory rate of 12–20 breaths per minute, breath sounds that are equal and clear bilaterally, and equal rise and fall of the chest are all parameters of normal respirations. (*) (FR7 p. 100; FRASA pp. 102–103)

88.

B. The size of the tongue in an infant proportionately is considerably larger than that of an adult. (*) (FR7 p. 108; FRASA p. 97)

89.

D. The narrowest portion of the upper airway in a patient under 10 years of age is at the cricoid ring, which is below the vocal cords. The narrowest portion of an adult's airway is at the level of the vocal cords. (*) (FR7 p. 108; FRASA p. 96)

90.

B. The infant is exhibiting signs of a partial airway obstruction. The stridorous respirations and the infant's color indicate oxygenation/ventilation is still occurring. (*) (FR7 p. 113; FRASA p. 135)

91.

C. If you suspect a partial airway obstruction, it is most important to keep your patient calm, instruct him or her to cough, and provide high-flow oxygen via a nonrebreather mask. (*) (FR7 p. 114; FRASA p. 136)

92.

C. In a complete airway obstruction, the patient will not be able to cough, whereas in the partial airway obstruction the patient will cough forcefully in an attempt to remove the object. (*) (FR7 p. 114; FRASA p. 136)

93.

A. Inspiration occurs due to the contraction of the diaphragm, which causes it to move downward, and the contraction of the intercostal muscles, which pulls the ribs outward, increasing thoracic cavity size and allowing air to rush in. (*) (FR7 p. 97; FRASA p. 96)

94.

D. Respiration is the molecular process of exchange of oxygen and carbon dioxide. Ventilation is the mechanical process of moving oxygen into the lungs and carbon dioxide out of the lungs. Oxygenation is the process of supplementing the oxygen content or providing oxygen therapy. (*) (FR7 p. 96; FRASA p. 56)

95.

D. The pharynx is a common passageway for food, water, and air. (*) (FR7 p. 99; FRASA p. 95)

96.

D. The occiput (back of the head) in the young child is disproportionately larger when compared with the child's body. The large occiput causes the flexion and leads to airway obstruction. To alleviate this problem in young children and infants, pad under the shoulders to bring the thorax up to the level of the head. (*) (FR7 p. 463; FRASA p. 97)

97.

C. The First Responder can only help administer the medication if it is in his or her protocol. In this situation explain your protocol to the family physician and defer further questioning to the medical director or on-line medical control. (*) (FR7 p. 5; FRASA p. 9)

98.

B. Asthma is an example of a lower-airway disease. Epiglottitis is a bacterial infection causing inflammation of the upper airway at the level of the epiglottis and subglottic area. (*) (FR7 p. 471, 473; FRASA pp. 259, 511)

99.

A. Patients that present in a tripod position are usually in severe respiratory distress. The tripod position is when patients sit upright and lean forward, supporting themselves with their arms, with elbows locked between their dangling legs. Occasionally you may find a severe respiratory distress patient lying supine or in a reclining position; these patients may be too exhausted to support themselves. (*) (FR7 p. 471; FRASA pp. 257–258)

100.

D. Apnea is the term used to describe the patient in respiratory arrest. Dyspnea is the term used to describe the patient who is having difficulty breathing. Bradypnea is the term used to describe the patient breathing at a rate that is less than the normal. Tachypnea describes the patient breathing faster than the normal respiratory rate. (*) (FR7 p. 471)

101.

B. The patient with cyanosis—a bluish-gray skin color on the neck or chest, an ominous sign of respiratory distress—requires immediate emergency intervention. The patient who can speak full sentences is most likely not in severe respiratory distress. The patient who can only speak one or two words in between breaths is in severe respiratory distress. Normal respiratory rates for children are 15–30 times each minute. It is normal for infants to use their abdominal muscles when breathing. (*) (FR7 p. 101; FRASA p. 106)

102.

D. Stridor is a high-pitched inspiratory sound that is caused by a narrowing of the upper airway. Stridor indicates that the airway is partially obstructed. Obstruction can be caused by a foreign body or swelling of the larynx. (*) (FR7 p. 113; FRASA p. 99)

103.

C. Hypotension, low blood pressure, is a late sign of respiratory distress in infants and children. When you encounter these late signs in the infant or child, you must immediately provide positive pressure ventilation. (*) (FR7 p. 473; FRASA p. 103)

104.

B. If you are unsure if the patient's condition warrants positive pressure ventilation, it is better to provide the ventilation than to delay the treatment. Delaying the treatment may worsen the respiratory condition and may lead to respiratory arrest and even death. Administering high-flow oxygen will not provide an adequate tidal volume. A nasopharyngeal airway alone will not help the patient with breathing difficulty. Placing the patient in the Trendelenburg (shock) position may worsen the patient's condition. (*) (FR7 p. 156; FRASA p. 102)

105.

A. Loss of muscle tone is a late sign of respiratory failure in an infant and must be managed immediately with positive pressure ventilation. Cyanosis of the extremities is an early sign of breathing difficulty in the infant. Tachycardia (fast heart rate) is an early sign, whereas bradycardia (slow heart rate) is a late sign of respiratory failure in the infant. Prolonged exhalation and nasal flaring are early signs of breathing difficulty. (*) (FR7 p. 473; FRASA p. 500)

106.

B. If the child will not tolerate a nonrebreather mask, you should have the parent hold the child and administer oxygen by holding the mask near but not on his face. Never withhold oxygen from any patient complaining of difficulty breathing. You should always speak to children softly; however, holding the mask on their face will only add to their stress. Always reassure your patient. Administering oxygen by nasal cannula is not appropriate in this situation. In addition, the liter flow is too high. (*) (FR7 p. 460; FRASA p. 510)

107.

C. Suspect the child has epiglottitis if he has a fever, sore throat, is sitting upright with his neck jutted out, and drooling. Epiglottitis is a true emergency and should be treated with high-flow oxygen and immediate transport to the hospital. You should consider ALS backup. Epiglottitis is a condition that causes the epiglottis to swell and the larynx to spasm, blocking the opening into the trachea. (*) (FR7 p. 471; FRASA p. 511)

108.

A. The barking-seal sound when the patient coughs is the hallmark sign of croup. Croup results in the swelling of the larynx, trachea, and bronchi. It is common for the condition to worsen at night. Apply oxygen, humidified if possible. (*) (FR7 p. 471; FRASA p. 510)

ALLERGIES AND ANAPHYLAXIS

109.

B. During an allergic reaction, sympathetic discharge in addition to the hypoxia will result in an increased heart rate. Urticaria is hives and pruritis is itching, the hallmark sign and symptom of allergic reaction. (*) (FR7 p. 261; FRASA p. 297)

110.

D. During an allergic reaction, the release of histamine and chemical mediators will cause edema (swelling) of the airway, increased mucus production, and bronchial smooth muscle constriction. (*) (FR7 pp. 261–262; FRASA p. 339)

111.

A. This patient is exhibiting signs and symptoms of a severe allergic reaction or anaphylaxis. This patient needs aggressive airway management and ventilatory support. Contacting ALS is important; however, you must keep airway and ventilation management as a primary concern. (*) (FR7 p. 262; FRASA p. 341)

112.

C. This patient is exhibiting signs of a mild reaction including the urticaria (hives) and pruritis (itching). This patient could advance to a more severe reaction, so constant reassessment of the airway, breathing, and circulation will be necessary. Without respiratory or cardiovascular system involvement,

there is no need to administer the epinephrine. Once it is evident that the respiratory system or cardiovascular system is involved, do not delay epinephrine administration. (*) (FRASA p. 341)

113.

A. A mild reaction can rapidly deteriorate to severe anaphylaxis involving severe respiratory compromise and cardiovascular collapse. (*) (FR7 p. 261; FRASA p. 338)

114.

A. Tachycardia (rapid heart rate) is a common sign even in a mild reaction. The tachycardia could be caused by the reaction or by the anxiety that the patient may be experiencing. Likewise, hives and flushed skin are found in mild reactions. Hypotension (low blood pressure) or evidence of poor perfusion (weak or absent peripheral pulses, decreased mental status) indicates cardiovascular compromise and the immediate need for epinephrine administration. (*) (FR7 p. 566; FRASA p. 341)

115.

B. Anaphylactic shock is characterized by cardiovascular collapse, which includes hypoperfusion and subsequent decreased level of consciousness; nasal flaring and tachypnea (rapid breathing) are signs of respiratory distress. Hemiparesis (weakness to one side of the body) is seen in stroke and head-injured patients. (*) (FR7 p. 262; FRASA pp. 338–339)

116.

C. The high-pitched sounds are stridorous respirations. Stridor indicates obstruction of the upper airway, usually from swelling of the larynx in anaphylaxis. The patient needs rapid and aggressive airway management. (*) (FR7 p. 113; FRASA p. 99)

117.

D. Closely assess the airway of the patient with an allergic reaction. Stridor or crowing sounds indicate significant swelling to the upper airway. A swollen tongue and additional signs of anaphylaxis may also be present. (*) (FR7 p. 262; FRASA p. 99)

118.

D. The use and administration of the epinephrine auto-injector requires either an off-line or on-line order from medical control. The medication is prescribed to the patient. It is an intramuscular injection. (*) (FR7 p. 262; FRASA p. 340)

119.

A. If the patient is suffering from a mild allergic reaction without respiratory compromise or signs of shock, do not administer epinephrine by auto-injector. Treatment includes high-flow oxygen, placing the patient in a position of comfort, completing your assessment, and transporting the patient. (*) (FR7 pp. 565–566; FRASA p. 341)

120.

A. You may need to force air past the swollen laryngeal tissue by providing positive pressure ventilation with a bag-valve-mask device or pocket-mask. Delivering ventilation may become difficult due to the high resistance. Deactivating the pop-off valve on the bag-valve-mask may help deliver adequate ventilation. The airway is compromised due to swelling of laryngeal tissue; thus inserting an airway adjunct, such as the oropharyngeal airway or nasopharyngeal airway, is of little help. (*) (FR7 p. 262; FRASA p. 341)

121.

C. The correct administration procedure for a prescribed epinephrine auto-injector is to 1) firmly place the auto-injector against the patient's thigh halfway between the knee and the waist, and 2) hold the injector in place until all of the drug is delivered. The injector will deliver the correct dose automatically if left in place until empty. (*) (FR7 pp. 566–567; FRASA pp. 340–341)

122.

C. The possible side effects to the administration of epinephrine are increased heart rate, pale skin, dizziness, chest pain, headache, nausea, vomiting, and anxiousness. You should advise your patient of these possible side effects when administering the drug. (*) (FR7 p. 566)

123.

A. There are no contraindications to administration of epinephrine by auto-injector in the severe anaphylactic patient. Never deliver a half dose to any patient, since the auto-injector will automatically deliver the adult a dose of 0.3 mg. Infants and children up to 66 lb. are prescribed epinephrine auto-injectors that deliver a dose of 0.15 mg. Stridor is an indication that the anaphylactic patient's airway is becoming compromised. Epinephrine by auto-injector is indicated. (*) (FR7 pp. 566–567; FRASA pp. 340–341)

124.

C. This patient is breathing inadequately and should receive immediate ventilatory support by positive pressure ventilation. (*) (FR7 pp. 259–260; FRASA p. 298)

125.

A. You should immediately obtain an order from medical direction to administer epinephrine by auto-injector. Delaying this action may cause the patient's condition to deteriorate further. Unless you have off-line orders for the administration of epinephrine by auto-injector, you must obtain the order prior to administering the drug. This patient is having a severe allergic reaction (anaphylaxis) and should receive epinephrine as quickly as possible. (*) (FR7 p. 566; FRASA pp. 9, 340)

126.

B. Common side effects of epinephrine are increased heart rate, pale skin, dizziness, chest pain, headache, nausea, vomiting, excitability, and anxiousness. (*) (FR7 p. 566)

127.

D. This patient is likely bleeding from veins. Bleeding from veins is typically a dark red, with a steady flow, and sometimes very heavy. Arterial bleeding usually is a brighter red, very heavy, and usually spurts with each contraction of the heart. Capillary bleeding is usually slow or oozing and the color is red; however, the red color is not as bright as arterial bleeding. (5-2.1) (FR7 pp. 287–288; FRASA p. 328)

128.

B. Arterial bleeding is sometimes difficult to control because of the higher pressure. Arterial blood is rich with oxygen, which causes the blood to be bright red. With each contraction of the heart, the artery spurts blood from the wound. Dark red with a steady flow describes venous bleeding. Oozing that usually clots spontaneously describes capillary bleeding. (5-2.1) (FR7 p. 287; FRASA p. 328)

129.

B. The patient is in shock from the blood loss. The breathing is adequate at 24 times a minute with good air exchange. Oxygen should be administered by nonrebreather mask at 15 lpm if available and your orders permit you to do so. You should continue with your assessment and treatment and call immediately for rapid transport by the EMS crew. (5-2.5) (FR7 pp. 305–306; FRASA p. 334)

130.

D. For bleeding in the upper extremity, the brachial artery pressure point would be used. For bleeding from the lower extremity, the femoral pressure point would be compressed. Use the heel of one hand or firm finger pressure for the femoral, and the fingertip pressure for the brachial. (5-2.2) (FR7 p. 293; FRASA pp. 331–332)

131.

C. A tourniquet is used only as a last resort to control bleeding. It should be made of a wide, bulky material that will not produce underlying soft-tissue injury. The tourniquet should be left uncovered and visible to medical personnel. Avoid placement directly over any joint. The tourniquet should be used after direct pressure and pressure points have failed to control bleeding. (5-2.2) (FR7 p. 295; FRASA p. 332)

132.

B. If direct pressure fails to control bleeding, you should next try direct pressure with elevation of the extremity. Do not elevate the extremity if a fracture is suspected. A tourniquet is reserved for severe uncontrolled bleeding. (5-2.2) (FR7 p. 289; FRASA p. 330)

133.

B. Internal bleeding may not be obvious. Always suspect internal bleeding if the patient presents with unexplained shock. Patients can lose large amounts of blood very rapidly internally. (5-2.4) (FR7 p. 302; FRASA p. 334)

134.

B. If you suspect the patient is in shock, you should establish a patent airway, manage the ventilation, administer oxygen, protect the spine while placing the patient in a supine position, and keep the patient warm. Once the EMS crew arrives, you should assist the EMS crew for immediate transport to the hospital. Do not delay transport to determine the exact cause of internal bleeding. Patients who are bleeding internally need immediate transport to the hospital where surgical procedures can be performed and blood can be administered. (5-2.5) (FR7 pp. 305–306; FRASA pp. 337–338)

135.

D. A rapid, thready, weak pulse is an early sign of possible internal bleeding and shock (hypoperfusion). Decreased blood pressure is a late sign of shock. The patient in shock will usually have a faster than normal breathing rate (tachypnea). A delayed capillary refill in the adult patient is usually greater than 2 seconds. (5-2.4) (FR7 p. 304; FRASA p. 335)

136.

C. The signs and symptoms of shock include restlessness; anxiety; pale, cool, clammy skin; weak pulse; increased pulse rate; increased respirations; decreasing blood pressure (late); dilated pupils; marked thirst; nausea, vomiting; and pallor. (5-2.4) (FR7 p. 304; FRASA p. 335)

137.

A. The outermost protective layer of skin is the epidermis. The dermis is the layer below the epidermis; this layer contains nerves, blood vessels, and sebaceous glands. The subcutaneous layer contains the fat and soft-tissue and is located below the dermis layer. (5-2.7) (FR7 p. 339; FRASA pp. 66, 387)

138.

C. Because of the obvious hazard of blood and body fluids associated with soft-tissue injuries, take body substance isolation precautions prior to patient contact. Be sure to wear gloves, face mask, and eye protection. (5-2.3) (FR7 p. 287; FRASA p. 334)

139.

A. An abrasion is caused by scraping of the outermost layer of the skin or epidermis. A puncture is a penetrating injury that results from a sharp, pointed object entering the soft-tissue. An avulsion results when a loose flap of skin or soft-tissue has been torn loose or pulled completely off. A laceration is a break in the skin of varying depth. (5-2.7) (FR7 p. 316; FRASA p. 350)

140.

B. An open wound to the chest is sealed with an occlusive or nonporous dressing to prevent air from entering the wound. An occlusive dressing is one that does not permit air to pass through it. Two examples are Vaseline gauze and plastic wrap. Plastic from an oxygen mask or abdominal dressing packaging could be used. The quickest occlusive dressing you can apply is your gloved hand. This will immediately seal the wound until a dressing can be applied. (5-2.9) (FR7 pp. 335–336; FRASA p. 353)

141.

C. By securing the occlusive dressing on three sides, trapped air within the chest will be permitted to escape while air outside the chest will not be permitted to enter the chest. Taping on three sides effectively makes the occlusive dressing a one-way (flapper) valve. (5-2.9) (FR7 p. 336; FRASA p. 353)

142.

D. The treatment for an open abdominal wound with an evisceration should include soaking a large, sterile, bulky dressing (trauma dressing) and covering the organs. Avoid any dressing that may adhere to the organs such as paper, toilet tissue, or paper towels. Place a nonporous dressing such as a large plastic wrap over the bulky dressing. This dressing helps to maintain the warmth of the internal organs and reduce moisture loss. The dressing may be held in place with a loose sheet or bandage. Position the patient in a position of comfort, with the hips and knees flexed. Do not attempt to replace the organs back in the abdominal cavity, and do not touch the organs. (5-2.10) (FR7 pp. 337–338; FRASA p. 378)

143.

C. Burns are classified as superficial or first degree (red skin), partial thickness or second degree (blisters), and full thickness or third degree burn (charring). Reddened skin that is painful, blistered, and weeping indicates a partial thickness burn. (5-2.13) (FR7 p. 341; FRASA p. 386)

144.

A. Burns that involve both the epidermis and portions of the dermis are known as partial thickness burns or second-degree burns. These burns can be caused by scalding and are painful. Superficial burns, also called first-degree burns, involve only the epidermis and are very painful. Full thickness burns involve all the layers of the skin (epidermis and dermis), and the subcutaneous layers. The tough and leathery dead soft-tissue formed by this burn is called an eschar. (5-2.13) (FR7 p. 341; FRASA p. 386)

145.

B. A partial thickness burn or a second-degree burn involves the epidermis and dermis. Partial thickness burns cause intense pain from nerve-ending damage and exposure. Partial thickness burns present as red, moist, and very painful with blister formation. (5-2.13) (FR7 p. 341; FRASA p. 386)

146.

A. A full thickness burn will appear dry, hard, tough, and leathery. It may appear white and waxy to dark brown or black and charred. The tough and leathery dead soft-tissue is called an eschar. (5-2.13) (FR7 p. 341; FRASA p. 386)

147.

B. The full thickness burn involves the epidermis, dermis, and subcutaneous layers of the skin. This type of burn often results in an eschar, leathery dead soft-tissue. The full thickness burn is also known as a third-degree burn and is the most severe or critical burn. (5-2.13) (FR7 p. 341; FRASA p. 386)

148.

A. Special management of a burn requires prevention of further contamination and injury to the burn area. Clothing that is adhering to the skin should be left intact. Removal could cause further tissue damage. Remove any jewelry from the hands. This will prevent restrictive blood flow from swelling that may occur. An exact calculation of the body surface area is not required. (5-2.13) (FR7 pp. 342–343; FRASA pp. 390–392)

149.

B. Never apply any type of ointment or lotion to the burns. Ointments may cause heat retention. Often hospital personnel must then remove the ointment by vigorous cleansing. You should cover the burns with a dry, sterile, particle-free burn dressing. Burn patients will often lose too much heat because of damage to their skin, which regulates temperature. Conserve heat loss by covering the patient with blankets. Administer high-flow oxygen by nonrebreather mask if the patient's breathing is adequate and you are able to do so according to your protocol. If breathing is inadequate, provide positive pressure ventilation. (5-2.13) (FR7 p. 343; FRASA pp. 389–391)

150.

A. If the bleeding continues to be severe and soaks through the dressing, remove the dressing, look for the vessel or site of bleeding, apply firm fingertip pressure to that area to stop the bleeding. Once the bleeding has been controlled, apply a sterile dressing. (5-2.2)

151.

C. You should never remove an impaled object unless it is impaled through the cheek or it is impaled in the chest and interferes with chest compressions while performing CPR. Removing impaled objects from areas other than the cheek can lead to further injury or even death. Impaled objects should be stabilized in place using bulky dressings and tape. (5-2.11) (FR7 p. 322; FRASA p. 354)

152.

B. Check for source and ground burn injury. Never touch a patient who is in contact with an electrical source. Never apply any type of burn ointment to any type of burn. An electrical burn patient requires oxygen via a nonrebreather mask at 15 lpm. Do not apply the AED until the patient is confirmed to be pulseless and apneic. (5-2.13) (FR7 p. 347; FRASA p. 394)

153.

C. Injury caused by an electrical burn can be quite extensive and involve many internal organs such as the heart, spleen, and lungs. If the source wound is on the left hand and the ground wound is on the feet, right hand, hip, knee, and so on, the path crosses the heart and other vital organs. Alternating current (AC) is a fibrillatory stimulus; thus, it has a tendency to put the heart in ventricular fibrillation. Therefore, electrical burn patients may be in cardiac arrest due to the electrical energy and may need CPR and defibrillation. Source and ground wounds are treated the same as other thermal burns. Because of the possible involvement of the heart and other vital organs, you should treat all patients with electrical burns as critical patients. (5-2.13) (FR7 p. 347; FRASA p. 393–394)

154.

D. The upper bone of the arm is called the humerus. The radius and ulna make up the lower portion of the arm. The scapula makes up the back of the shoulder. (5-3.1) (FR7 p. 355; FRASA p. 466)

155.

D. Before and after splinting, check for pulse, motor function, and sensation in the injured extremity. This should be evaluated every 15 minutes after applying the splint. This ensures that the splint is not impairing circulation. (5-3.3) (FR7 p. 368; FRASA p. 465)

156.

A. Elevating this patient's extremity is not performed because of the possibility that he suffered a spinal injury. You should apply cold packs to decrease pain and edema (swelling) and dress any open wounds. You should assess the patient's motor, sensation, and distal pulse before and after the splint is applied. (5-3.3) (FR7 p. 403; FRASA p. 465)

157.

D. When a joint is injured, you should immobilize the bones above and below the affected joint. When a bone is injured, you should immobilize the joints above and below the affected bone. (5-3.3) (FR7 p. 380; FRASA p. 467)

158.

C. If the extremity is cyanotic and pulseless, you may make one attempt to align the extremity by applying gentle traction to the extremity before splinting. If the pain, resistance, or crepitus increase, you must stop. Do not try to align a wrist, elbow, knee, hip, or shoulder because of major nerves and blood vessels that lie close to these joints. (5-3.3) (FR7 p. 369; FRASA p. 465)

159.

C. Never intentionally replace a protruding bone into the extremity because further tissue damage may result. You should assess the distal pulse and motor and sensory function before and after the splint is applied. To effectively immobilize a long bone, you must immobilize the joint above and below the injured bone. Never try to align an injury that involves the wrist, elbow, knee, hip, or shoulder; doing so may cause more injury. (5-3.3) (FR7 pp. 369–370; FRASA p. 465)

160.

B. The nervous system that consists of the brain and the spinal cord is the central nervous system. The peripheral nervous system consists of nerves located outside the brain and spinal cord. The voluntary nervous system influences the activity of the voluntary muscles and moves the body. The autonomic nervous system influences the activity of involuntary muscles and glands and regulates the heart rate and breathing. (5-3.7) (FR7 p. 61; FRASA pp. 59, 61)

161.

B. The cranium consists of fused bones and is referred to as the skull. Because the skull consists of rigid bone, it protects the brain from injury. (5-3.7) (FR7 p. 396; FRASA p. 421)

162.

C. A rare sign of spinal injury is an obvious deformity of the spine. This is usually found when palpating the spine. More common signs or symptoms of spinal injury are loss of motor function (patient unable to move) or loss of sensory function (unable to feel) below the site of spinal injury. (5-3.6) (FR7 pp. 400–401; FRASA p. 442)

163.

D. Patients with possible spine injuries must be managed carefully. Improper handling can cause further injury or death. When you suspect a patient may have a spine injury, you must open and maintain the airway using the jaw-thrust maneuver. Cervical traction is not used in the prehospital setting. This technique can cause further injury including paralysis. Lateral-lift or head-tilt maneuvers will compromise the spine and may cause further injury. (5-3.8) (FR7 p. 403; FRASA pp. 442, 99)

164.

C. Spinal immobilization and placement on a long spine board are ideally performed by four rescuers. One maintains cervical spine stabilization, and three rescuers perform the logroll. A fifth rescuer can be used to place the board under the patient. (5-3.5) (FR7 pp. 81–82; FRASA p. 444)

165.

B. Measure the distance from an imaginary line from the top of the shoulder to the bottom of the jaw line. Use your fingers to measure the distance. (5-3.5) (FR7 p. 87; FRASA p. 444)

166.

A. When you encounter a standing patient with a possible spine injury, you must place the patient onto the board, using the standing long board technique. This technique consists of placing the board behind the patient and lowering the patient from the standing position. You must maintain control of the patient's head and cervical spine with manual stabilization and the use of a cervical collar. When lowering the patient, support the patient by placing a rescuer at the side of the board to support the patient under the arms. All of the other techniques will compromise the spine and possibly cause further injury to the patient. (5-3.6)

167.

C. A short spine board or a vest-type device is used to immobilize a patient who is found in a seated position. (5-3.6) (FR7 p. 83; FRASA pp. 445, 449)

168.

B. This patient should be extricated using the rapid-extrication technique. The rapid-extrication technique should be used in the following situations: 1) the scene is not safe (due to fire, explosion, chemical spill, etc.); 2) the patient's condition is so critical and unstable that you need to move and transport the patient immediately; and 3) the patient blocks your access to a second, more seriously injured patient. (5-3.5) (FR7 pp. 70–71; FRASA p. 447)

169.

B. Rapid extrication is indicated if the scene is not safe or if the patient's condition is unstable. A stable patient who blocks the access to a second patient who is critically injured may also require rapid extrication. A stable patient does not generally require rapid extrication. (5-3.5) (FR7 pp. 70–71; FRASA p. 447)

170.

C. If the patient is in cardiac arrest, you must remove the helmet. You should also remove the helmet if the helmet interferes with proper spinal immobilization; the helmet does not fit well and allows excessive movement; the helmet interferes with your ability to adequately manage the airway or breathing; or the helmet interferes with your ability to assess or reassess the airway or breathing. (5-3.8) (FR7 pp. 406–407; FRASA p. 449)

171.

A. The two basic helmet types are the sports helmet and the motorcycle helmet. (5-3.8) (FR7 pp. 406–407; FRASA p. 449)

172.

B. The football helmet should be left in place unless there is a life threat that requires its removal. The player's shoulder pads and helmet create a neutral alignment of the spine. Removal of the helmet causes the head to flex. (5-3.8) (FR7 p. 407; FRASA p. 449)

173.

C. The patient is complaining of cervical spine pain and was involved in an incident with a significant mechanism of injury. Immediately provide cervical spine stabilization and initiate a standing takedown. Do not allow the patient to walk, sit, or lie down. (5-3.8) (FR7 p. 406; FRASA p. 442)

174.

A. She may be exhibiting early signs and symptoms of a head injury. It is important to immediately conduct an initial assessment to ensure she has an open airway and adequate breathing, and then to assess her perfusion status. (5-3.8) (FR7 p. 399; FRASA p. 421)

175.

B. The level of consciousness is continuing to decline. The airway apparently is partially obstructed from the tongue. As the level of consciousness continues to decline, the muscles continue to relax, and the patient is unable to maintain her own airway. You must reposition the airway using a jaw-thrust and insert a mechanical airway if the patient continues to present with a partially obstructed airway. (5-3.8) (FR7 p. 399; FRASA p. 421)

176.

D. Burns that involve all layers of the skin including tissue below the subcutaneous layer are classified as full thickness burns. Full thickness burns may appear dark brown, black, waxy, dry, hard, leathery, or white. Often the patient with a full thickness burn will experience little pain due to the nerve endings being exposed by the burn injury. (5-2.13) (FR7 p. 341; FRASA p. 386)

177.

D. Any burns that encircle a body part, upper extremities, legs, chest, or neck are classified as a critical burn. Burns also to hands, face, feet, and genitalia are considered critical. (5-2.13) (FR7 p. 341; FRASA p. 389)

178.

A. You should apply dry sterile dressings after you remove clothing and initially cool the burn site with sterile water. You should never apply a burn ointment or salve, break blisters, or attempt to remove any burned skin. Ice is not applied to a burn because it will promote hypothermia (general cooling of the body), and it could lead to direct tissue damage if applied directly to the damaged skin and for too long of a period. (5-3.13) (FR7 pp. 342–343; FRASA pp. 389–390)

179.

D. Once you have determined the scene is safe, you must first conduct an initial assessment and manage life threats to the airway, breathing, and circulation. Thus, you must suction the airway, insert an oropharyngeal airway, and begin positive pressure ventilation in this patient. (5-3-8) (FR7 pp. 125, 129, 399; FRASA pp. 122, 421)

180.

C. Flexion of the extremities and arching of the back on painful stimulation are indications of an injury to the upper brain stem. This is a form of non-purposeful movement and is also known as decorticate posturing. (5-3.7) (FR7 p. 397; FRASA p. 422)

181.

B. The best treatment that could be provided to this head-injured patient is to establish and maintain a patent airway and provide effective ventilation. If possible, supplemental oxygen should be connected to the ventilation device. Patients with a head injury may also have suffered a spinal injury; thus, you would keep the patient in a supine (flat on his back face up) position and maintain manual spinal stabilization. (5-3.8) (FR7 p. 399; FRASA p. 421)

6 Childbirth and Children

module objectives

Questions in this module relate to D.O.T. objectives 6-1.1 to 6-2.10.

CHILDBIRTH AND CHILDREN 6-1

1. In a normal pregnancy, which female reproductive organ houses the developing fetus until the child is born?
   A. cervix
   B. placenta
   C. uterus
   D. fallopian tubes

2. This is the sole organ through which the fetus receives oxygen and nourishment and discharges carbon dioxide and other waste products.
   A. amniotic sac
   B. placenta
   C. cervix
   D. fallopian tubes

3. You arrive at the local doctor's office and find your patient lying on the bed, moaning in pain. The nurse tells you that the patient is 9 months pregnant and that she is having contractions 2 minutes apart and lasting 45 seconds. The nurse adds that the patient has the need to move her bowels. As your partner prepares the obstetric kit, your next immediate action should be to:
   A. wait for the EMS crew to transport because her labor may last for hours.
   B. examine her vaginal area for crowning.
   C. place the patient in the first response vehicle and begin transport rapidly.
   D. place the patient's legs together to delay the delivery.

4. When preparing to cut the umbilical cord, approximately how far from the infant's abdomen should the first clamp be placed on the umbilical cord?
   A. 12 inches
   B. 10 inches
   C. 6 inches
   D. 2 inches

5. What are the minimum requirements for body substance isolation when you are preparing to perform a delivery?
   A. gloves, eye protection, and head nets
   B. mask, gloves, and foot protectors
   C. gown, gloves, and mask
   D. mask, gown, gloves, and eye protection

6. Approximately how far from the first cord clamp should the second cord clamp be placed on the umbilical cord?
   A. 1 inch
   B. 3 inches
   C. 6 inches
   D. 10 inches

7. The treatment sequence for neonatal resuscitation is:
   A. position, warm, dry, suction, tactile stimuli, oxygen, BVM, chest compressions.
   B. dry, warm, position, stimulate, suction, oxygen, BVM, chest compressions.
   C. dry, warm, position, suction, stimulate, oxygen, chest compressions, BVM.
   D. dry, warm, position, suction, stimulate, oxygen, BVM, chest compressions.

8. What are the indications for performing chest compressions in the newborn?
   A. when the blood pressure drops below 90 mmHg
   B. when the newborn's pulse drops below 130 bpm for over 1 minute
   C. when the heart rate drops below 60 bpm
   D. when the heart rate falls below 100 bpm

9. A foul-smelling, greenish-brown, thick, viscous fluid that may be present in the amniotic fluid is:

    A. afterbirth.

    B. meconium.

    C. dried blood.

    D. the bloody show.

10. The presence of meconium in the amniotic fluid is usually an indication of:

    A. precipitative delivery.

    B. poor prenatal care.

    C. fetal distress.

    D. congenital deformities.

11. When you suspect meconium in the amniotic sac or in the infant's airway, you should:

    A. stimulate the infant immediately to allow full expansion of the infant's lungs to prevent fetal hypoxia.

    B. immediately warm and stimulate the patient because the meconium can depress the infant's ability to warm itself.

    C. help stimulate the baby's cough reflex to allow removal of the meconium from the lungs.

    D. immediately suction the airway first before any other treatment, including stimulation.

12. When the head of the newborn is delivered, you should gently place a gloved hand over the head to prevent an explosive delivery during a forceful contraction and tearing the perineum. The perineum is the:

    A. area between the vagina and the anus.

    B. organ that the umbilical cord is attached to.

    C. opening of the uterus.

    D. lateral aspects of the vagina.

13. You are delivering a baby and notice a thick, viscous fluid all over the baby and a foul smell. Your immediate reaction and treatment should be to:

    A. finish the delivery and activate ALS immediately.

    B. begin to suction the baby's mouth and nose immediately.

    C. wait for the placenta to deliver before you begin cleaning the baby off.

    D. do nothing because this is a normal event.

14. You delivered a baby and are providing positive pressure ventilation. You reassess the baby and determine that the infant's heart rate is 138 bpm, respirations are 38/minute with good chest rise, and the skin is pink. You should:

    A. continue to ventilate because the vitals signs are still not adequate.

    B. continue to ventilate but at a rate of 20 per minute.

    C. decrease the ventilation rate to 12 per minute.

    D. stop providing ventilation and reassess the respirations and heart rate in 1 minute.

15. What is the compression-to-ventilation ratio for infant CPR?

    A. 15 compressions to 1 ventilation per minute

    B. 30 compressions to 5 ventilations per minute

    C. 30 compressions to 2 ventilations per minute

    D. 60 compressions to 10 ventilations per minute

16. The correct depth for chest compressions in a newborn is:

    A. one-half the depth of the chest.

    B. $\frac{1}{4}$ to $\frac{3}{4}$ inch in depth.

    C. $\frac{1}{4}$ to $\frac{1}{2}$ inch in depth.

    D. one-third to one-half the depth of the chest.

17. You begin to assist ventilations in a newborn. How often should you reassess your treatment and the patient's response?

    A. every 30 seconds

    B. every minute

    C. every 2 minutes

    D. every 3–5 minutes

18. The condition that may result when the combined weight of the enlarged uterus and fetus compresses the vena cava and reduces the blood return to the heart while the patient is lying on her back is called:

    A. gravid uterus syndrome.

    B. hypertensive uterine syndrome.

    C. fatal hypoperfusion syndrome.

    D. supine hypotensive syndrome.

19. Vaginal bleeding should be managed by:

    A. placing the patient in a Fowler's position.

    B. placing a pad over the vaginal opening.

    C. packing pads into the vagina to control excessive blood loss.

    D. placing additional pads on top of blood-soaked pads.

20. Expulsion of fetal tissue that results in termination of the pregnancy is termed:

    A. placenta previa.

    B. abruptio placenta.

    C. breech presentation.

    D. spontaneous abortion.

21. When performing a normal delivery:

    A. put on eye protection only when preparing to deliver.

    B. hold the mother's legs together to prevent an explosive delivery.

    C. always take the maximum body substance isolation precautions.

    D. it is acceptable to allow the mother to use the bathroom when she has the urge to defecate.

22. Recommended equipment for a sterile obstetric kit includes all of the following except:

    A. bulb syringe.

    B. sanitary napkins.

    C. bag-valve-mask.

    D. cord clamps.

23. As soon as the head is delivered:

    A. quickly provide aggressive uterine massage.

    B. suction the mouth first and then the nose.

    C. begin ventilation.

    D. suction the nose first and then the mouth.

24. During delivery of the infant's head, excessive pressure should be:

    A. used to remove the cord from around the infant's neck.

    B. used to puncture the amniotic sac.

    C. used over the perineum to reduce the risk of tears.

    D. avoided over the fontanel area of the head.

25. Following delivery of the infant's head, you should immediately:

    A. create a sterile field around the vaginal opening.

    B. determine if the umbilical cord is around the neck of the baby.

    C. record the time of delivery on the medical report.

    D. deeply suction the back of the infant's mouth.

26. Blood loss of up to _____ cc is normal during childbirth and typically well tolerated by the mother.

    A. 100

    B. 300

    C. 500

    D. 700

27. Uterine massage is performed to:
    A. increase the uterus size by smooth muscle relaxation.
    B. stimulate milk production.
    C. reduce uterine contractions.
    D. contract the uterine smooth muscle.

28. In a multiple birth (twins, triplets):
    A. each infant always has its own placenta.
    B. each infant always shares a placenta.
    C. infants may have their own placenta or share one.
    D. the placenta is abnormally large.

29. In multiple births, about _____ of the deliveries of the second infant will be breech.
    A. 75 percent
    B. 66 percent
    C. 50 percent
    D. 33 percent

30. Place in the correct sequence the following steps for treatment of the patient with an injury to the external female genitalia.
    1. Ensure airway, breathing, and circulation.
    2. Provide transportation.
    3. Care for bleeding from the vagina.
    4. Administer oxygen.

    A. 1, 3, 4, 2
    B. 3, 1, 4, 2
    C. 1, 4, 3, 2
    D. 4, 1, 3, 2

31. You have responded to a vehicle accident. Upon arrival you observe a pregnant patient who is the unrestrained driver of the vehicle. She was involved in a low-speed accident in a parking lot at the grocery store. She tells you that she struck the back end of a car while traveling about 15 miles per hour. She is about a week from her due date. The patient refuses treatment. When assessing her for evidence of bleeding from trauma, you should:
    A. expect the blood pressure to fall quickly.
    B. not bother checking peripheral perfusion.

    C. realize that signs of shock may be subtle and the patient can deteriorate quickly.
    D. rely only on a decrease in heart rate as the best evidence of blood loss.

32. The patient in question 31 begins complaining of lower abdominal pain. Which of the following questions would be least important when obtaining a history of the present illness from this patient?
    A. How intense is the pain?
    B. What is the quality of the pain?
    C. Is the pain constant?
    D. Do you take any over-the-counter medications?

33. A pregnant patient in her third trimester complains of intermittent abdominal pain that occurs about every 2 minutes and lasts for about 1 minute. The patient's abdomen is very rigid on palpation. The patient tells you that she needs to use the bathroom. You should:
    A. allow the patient to use the bathroom.
    B. have the patient rest in bed for a few days.
    C. evaluate the patient for signs of crowning.
    D. place the patient in a prone position.

34. Your initial suctioning of a newborn's mouth and nose with a bulb syringe should be performed:
    A. immediately following the cutting of the umbilical cord.
    B. as soon as the entire delivery of the infant is completed.
    C. as soon as the head is delivered.
    D. directly after the torso is delivered.

35. When initially removing fluids from a newborn's airway during the birth process, you should:
    A. place the bulb syringe into position and then compress the bulb.
    B. suction the mouth first and then suction the nose.
    C. advance the tip of the bulb syringe until it touches the back of the pharynx.
    D. stimulate the newborn prior to removing fluid with the bulb syringe.

36. You are treating a nontrauma pregnant patient who is close to full term. To prevent hypotensive syndrome, you should:

    A. place the patient on her back with knees bent.

    B. manually displace the uterus to the right.

    C. place the patient in a supine position.

    D. place the patient in a supine position with her right hip elevated.

37. Which emergency medical treatment is inappropriate when assisting the delivery of a newborn?

    A. Tear the amniotic sac with your fingers if it has not ruptured during crowning.

    B. If bleeding appears heavy after delivery, massage the mother's abdomen.

    C. Place the first umbilical clamp approximately 6 inches from the infant.

    D. Apply pressure to the fontanel to prevent an explosive delivery.

38. Which statement is correct regarding the delivery of the placenta?

    A. When the placenta appears in the vaginal opening, grasp it and guide it from the vagina.

    B. Pull the placenta and all attached membranes from the vagina.

    C. Remain on scene until the placenta and attached membranes are delivered.

    D. Place the placenta and membranes in a biohazard bag and dispose of properly.

39. Your pregnant patient is in active labor, and you encounter a limb presentation in which the fetus's arm is protruding from the vagina. You should:

    A. place the mother in a head-down supine position with her pelvis elevated.

    B. gently pull the limb until the fetus is in the proper position for delivery.

    C. place your gloved hand into the vagina and maneuver the fetus into position.

    D. push the limb back into the vagina while pushing on the mother's abdomen.

40. Which of the following indicates that an infant is premature?

    A. The infant has coarse hair.

    B. There are many creases across the sole of the foot.

    C. There is no cartilage in the infant's outer ear.

    D. The infant weighs $6\frac{1}{2}$ pounds at birth.

41. You are caring for a newborn who was born during the 36th week of pregnancy. Which of the following emergency treatments is a priority for this patient?

    A. Provide high-flow oxygen by nonrebreather mask.

    B. Place the infant in warmed blankets.

    C. Suction secretions with a tonsil tip catheter.

    D. Cover the infant except for the head.

SCENARIO

Questions 42–44 refer to the following scenario:

You and your partner Jim are refueling your vehicle when you are dispatched for a woman in active labor. You quickly secure the fuel pump and respond to the emergency. On arrival at the scene, you find a 23-year-old woman lying supine on her bed. The amniotic sac has ruptured and she feels as if she must push. Jim quickly inspects the vagina for crowning and finds the pulsating umbilical cord protruding.

42. In which position should you and Jim place this patient?

    A. prone with chest elevated with pillows

    B. supine with the hips elevated with pillows

    C. semi-sitting with knees bent slightly

    D. lying flat on right side with knees bent

43. On reassessment, you notice the baby's head appears to be pushing against the pulsating umbilical cord. You should immediately:
    A. place a gloved hand into the vagina and gently push the head back and away from the cord.
    B. with your gloved hand, gently pull the cord away from the baby's head.
    C. with your gloved hand, gently push the pulsating cord back into the vagina.
    D. place a gloved hand into the vagina and push the vaginal wall away from the cord.

44. After applying pressure against the fetal head, you observe that the mother is breathing 42 times per minute with shallow breathing. You should immediately:
    A. provide oxygen by nasal cannula at 6 lpm.
    B. provide oxygen by nonrebreather mask at 15 lpm.
    C. open the airway and begin positive pressure ventilation.
    D. place the patient supine and elevate her right hip.

INFANTS AND CHILDREN 6-2

45. A child up to 12 months of age is referred to as a(n):
    A. preschooler.
    B. toddler.
    C. neonate.
    D. infant.

46. Which pediatric age group does not like to be touched, separated from parents, or have clothing removed, and fears needles?
    A. infant
    B. toddler
    C. preschooler
    D. school-age

47. Which pediatric age group uses concrete thinking skills and believes he or she is invincible?
    A. toddler
    B. preschooler
    C. school-age
    D. adolescent

48. Which anatomical or physiological difference in the infant and child patient is **correct** as compared to the adult?
    A. An infant's rib cage is less pliable, resulting in more injury.
    B. Infants have a faster metabolic rate that uses oxygen at a faster rate.
    C. Children's heads are proportionally smaller, leading to more head injuries.
    D. A child's skin surface is small compared to body mass, causing hypothermia.

49. Which statement is **incorrect** relating to anatomical differences between the adult and infant and child?
    A. A child's skin surface area is large when compared to body mass.
    B. Children's heads are proportionally larger than those of adults.
    C. Infants have proportionally larger tongues than those of adults.
    D. Children have a larger circulating blood volume than that of adults.

50. An infant or child responds to illness or injury differently than an adult. Which of the following statements best describes a typical **adult's** response to illness or injury?
    A. While crying, the patient says, "It hurts bad."
    B. "Don't touch me!"
    C. "I want to go home!"
    D. "My left arm hurts just below the elbow."

51. The leading medical cause of cardiac arrest in the infant or child patient is:
    A. cardiovascular disease.
    B. drowning or near drowning.
    C. respiratory failure.
    D. seizures.

52. All of the following are signs of early respiratory distress in the infant or child patient **except:**
    A. retractions between the ribs.
    B. nasal flaring.
    C. bradypnea (slow respiratory rate).
    D. increase in respiratory rate.

53. An infant or child patient who presents with agonal respirations and limp muscle tone, and is unresponsive with a slower-than-normal heart rate, is in:
    A. respiratory arrest.
    B. decompensated respiratory failure.
    C. compensated respiratory failure.
    D. early respiratory failure.

54. Which of the following signs, in addition to the signs of early respiratory distress (compensated respiratory failure), would indicate your infant or child patient is in respiratory failure?
    A. neck muscle use
    B. "see-saw" respirations
    C. decreased muscle tone
    D. nasal flaring on inspiration

55. An alert, crying child presents with stridor, is pink in color, and is displaying retractions of the chest muscles. The mother believes that "something is caught in his throat." The potential problem presented is a _____ and requires you to _____.
    A. partial airway obstruction, place the child in a position of comfort and instruct the child to cough forcefully
    B. partial airway obstruction, administer five back blows and five chest thrusts

C. complete airway obstruction, administer five abdominal thrusts
D. complete airway obstruction, administer five back blows and five abdominal thrusts

56. Which treatment is indicated for an 8-month-old infant with a complete airway obstruction?
    A. head-up position while delivering abdominal thrusts
    B. head-up position while delivering chest thrusts and back blows
    C. head-down position while delivering abdominal thrusts
    D. head-down position while delivering back slaps and chest thrust

57. While suctioning an infant patient, the suction should be limited to:
    A. 5–10 seconds.
    B. 10–15 seconds.
    C. 15–20 seconds.
    D. 20–30 seconds.

58. Infants and children require a respiratory tidal volume of _____ ml/kg with each breath.
    A. 5–10
    B. 10–15
    C. 15–20
    D. 20–25

59. An unresponsive child with facial trauma requires airway management. Which procedure should be avoided?
    A. insertion of an oropharyngeal airway
    B. insertion of a nasopharyngeal airway
    C. manual jaw-thrust technique
    D. moving the head into a neutral in-line position

60. An early indication of severe shock (hypoperfusion) in children is _____ because their _____, which helps to maintain the blood pressure.
    A. common, blood vessels constrict
    B. uncommon, blood vessels constrict

C. common, blood volume increases

D. uncommon, respiratory rate increases

61. All of the following are signs of shock (hypoperfusion) in the child **except:**

    A. pale, cool skin.

    B. bounding, peripheral pulse.

    C. absence of tears when crying.

    D. decreased urination.

62. A normal temperature for an infant or child is:

    A. 102° F.

    B. 100° F.

    C. 98° F.

    D. 95° F.

63. The least common cause of shock (hypoperfusion) in a child is:

    A. cardiac events.

    B. diarrhea.

    C. dehydration.

    D. vomiting.

64. All of the following are signs of adequate perfusion in an infant or child patient **except:**

    A. capillary refill less than 2 seconds.

    B. warm hands and feet.

    C. altered mental status.

    D. normal urinary output.

65. You are treating an 8-year-old patient. Which of the following signs or symptoms would indicate hypoperfusion (shock) in this patient?

    A. peripheral pulse of 80 bpm

    B. bounding peripheral pulse

    C. capillary refill of less than 2 seconds

    D. rapid respiratory rate

66. Which of the following is a common cause of seizures in children but **not** in adults?

    A. epilepsy

    B. hypoglycemia

    C. overdose

    D. fever

67. A seizure in an infant or child that lasts longer than 15 minutes or recurs without a recovery period is called:

    A. grand mal activity.

    B. mega-seizure activity.

    C. multi-seizure activity.

    D. status epilepticus.

68. You are treating a child who was an unrestrained front-seat passenger in a motor vehicle crash. Your patient is most likely to suffer:

    A. spinal and lower-extremity injuries.

    B. chest and abdominal injuries.

    C. upper-extremity and spinal injuries.

    D. head and neck injuries.

69. The leading cause of death of children 1–14 years of age is:

    A. trauma.

    B. cardiovascular disease.

    C. drowning.

    D. asthma.

70. When providing positive pressure ventilation to the injured child, special care must be taken to avoid _____, which can be reduced by using _____ during ventilation.

    A. gastric distention, cricoid pressure

    B. oropharyngeal airway placement, manual airway techniques

    C. head movement, the head-tilt chin-lift

    D. excessive ventilatory pressures, an oropharyngeal airway

71. Which of the following is **not** a general indicator of child abuse?

    A. rapid reporting of injuries

    B. lack of adult supervision

    C. injuries don't match mechanism

    D. a fearful child

72. In most child-abuse cases, the child suffers from:

    A. physical abuse.

    B. emotional abuse.

    C. sexual abuse.

    D. physical, emotional, and sexual abuse.

73. Which statement is **incorrect** relating to the care of the potential child-abuse patient?
    A. Use subjective information in your patient care report.
    B. Do not make accusatory statements to the parents.
    C. Do not allow the child to be alone with the suspected abuser.
    D. Know the abuse-reporting law in your community.

74. What action is frequently required following a traumatic-child or -infant call?
    A. meeting with local law enforcement personnel
    B. extensive cleaning of emergency vehicle
    C. debriefing of parents and friends
    D. critical-incident stress debriefing assistance

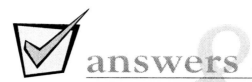

answers & rationales

Following each rationale, you will find a reference to the corresponding D.O.T. objective. A rationale marked with an asterisk denotes material supplemental to the First Responder curriculum. Also included after each rationale are references to where the question topic may be covered in Brady First Responder textbooks. **"FR7" refers to** *First Responder,* **7e** (Bergeron, Bizjak, Krause, Le Baudour). **"FRASA" refers to** *First Responder: A Skills Approach,* **7e** (Limmer, Karren, Hafen).

CHILDBIRTH AND CHILDREN 6-1

1.
C. The uterus is a hollow muscle that houses the fetus until birth. (6-1.1) (FR7 p. 422; FRASA p. 477)

2.
B. The placenta is the organ that allows for nourishment of the fetus. (6-1.1) (FR7 p. 423; FRASA p. 477)

3.
B. Contractions that are occurring every 2 minutes or less and lasting 30–90 seconds, along with the patient's urgency to move her bowels (caused by the baby placing pressure on the rectum) are all signs that the child is ready to deliver. In any patient in active labor, it is necessary to check the vaginal area for crowning. This will determine the urgency of the labor and the need for delivery. (6-1.3) (FR7 p. 423; FRASA p. 479)

4.
C. The first clamp should be placed approximately 6 inches from the infant's abdomen. (6-1.6) (FR7 p. 432; FRASA p. 485)

5.
D. The birthing process involves many different body fluids, so the minimum body substance isolation precautions include mask, gown, gloves, and eye protection. (6-1.5) (FR7 p. 425; FRASA p. 481)

6.
B. The second clamp should be placed approximately 3 inches from the first clamp. (6-1.6) (FR7 p. 432; FRASA p. 485)

7.
D. The inverted pyramid for neonatal resuscitation involves drying, warming, suctioning, stimulating, providing blow-by oxygen, positive pressure ventilation, and then CPR. (6-19.10) (FR7 pp. 435–437; FRASA p. 484)

8.
C. If at any time the infant's heart rate drops below 60 bpm, chest compressions should be initiated. (6-1.10) (FR7 p. 436; FRASA p. 484)

9.
B. Meconium is fecal matter excreted by the infant usually due to distress during the delivery. Meconium aspiration carries a high mortality rate. If meconium is noted in the amniotic fluid, be sure to suction all of it clear from the oropharynx and nasopharynx. (6-1.10) (FR7 p. 443; FRASA p. 482)

10.
C. Meconium is usually a result of fetal distress caused by decreased oxygen to the fetus or a prolonged labor. (6-1.10) (FR7 p. 443; FRASA p. 482)

11.
D. Immediate suctioning of the newborn's airway takes precedence over all other procedures. (6-1.10) (FR7 p. 443; FRASA p. 482)

12.
A. The perineum is the area of tissue between the vagina and anus. This area can tear during a rapid delivery or when the infant is large. The perineum is the area where the episiotomy is done to facilitate delivery. (6-1.1) (FR7 p. 431)

13.
B. The foul smell is from the meconium, and the airway needs to be suctioned immediately. (6-1.10) (FR7 p. 443; FRASA p. 482)

14.
D. Infants may respond very favorably to short periods of ventilation. Once the newborn's heart rate, ventilation, and oxygen status are determined to be adequate, stop ventilation and continuously reassess the newborn. (6-1.10) (FR7 pp. 435–436; FRASA p. 484)

15.

A. The ratio for infant CPR is 30 compressions to 2 ventilations. (6-1.10)

16.

D. The correct depth is one-third to one-half the depth of the chest. (6-1.10)

17.

A. Reassess the infant every 30 seconds to see if the infant is responding to the treatment or is getting worse. (6-1.10) (FR7 p. 435; FRASA p. 484)

18.

D. A condition that occurs during the third trimester of pregnancy is called supine hypotensive syndrome. It occurs as a result of the combined weight of the fetus and uterus compressing the inferior vena cava in the abdominal cavity. This pressure obstructs the blood return to the heart via the inferior vena cava while the patient is lying supine. This obstruction causes the blood pressure to decrease and the patient to faint or feel lightheaded. (*) (FR7 p. 448; FRASA p. 480)

19.

B. Save any passed tissue for transport with the EMS crew and examination by hospital personnel. Packing sanitary napkins or pads into the vagina is inappropriate. If a pad becomes soaked with blood, it should be replaced. If bleeding is excessive, it can become a life-threatening emergency. Carefully evaluate the patient for signs and symptoms of shock. (6-1.9) (FR7 p. 432; FRASA p. 485)

20.

D. A miscarriage or spontaneous abortion can occur for many different reasons. Fetal tissue is normally passed through the vagina. Signs and symptoms include cramp-like lower abdominal pain, moderate to severe vaginal bleeding, and passage of tissue or blood clots. (6-1.2) (FR7 p. 442; FRASA p. 486)

21.

C. Body substance isolation precautions are required, including mask, gown, and eye protection. Never hold the mother's legs together to delay delivery. Do not allow the mother to use the bathroom. This is likely a result of the infant's head moving down the birth canal and pressing against the patient's rectum and may result in the mother delivering the fetus in the toilet. (6-1.5) (FR7 p. 427; FRASA p. 481)

22.

C. Recommended equipment for an obstetric kit includes surgical scissors, hemostats or cord clamps, umbilical tape, bulb syringe, towels, gauze sponges, sterile gloves, infant blanket, individually wrapped sanitary napkins, large plastic bag, and germicidal wipes. A BVM is not a part of the obstetric kit. (6-1.4) (FR7 p. 425; FRASA p. 481)

23.

B. As soon as the head is delivered, support the head and suction. Suction the mouth first and then the nose. Compress the bulb syringe and suction two or three times to remove fluid and secretions. Insert the tip 1.0–1.5 inches into the infant's mouth. Avoid touching the back of the mouth with the tip of the bulb syringe. (6-1.7) (FR7 p. 430; FRASA p. 483)

24.

D. Excessive pressure should be avoided over the fontanel or soft spot. Excessive pressure should not be used for any delivery procedure. (6-1.7) (FR7 p. 428; FRASA pp. 482–483)

25.

B. Upon delivery of the head, you should immediately check the position of the umbilical cord and determine if the cord is wrapped around the infant's neck. The creation of a sterile field should have been accomplished prior to the delivery of the head. Avoid deep suctioning of the infant's mouth as this may result in bradycardia (slow heart rate). You will have plenty of time after delivery to record the time of birth. (6-1.7) (FR7 p. 431; FRASA p. 483)

26.

C. Up to 500 cc is normal. If blood loss is excessive, administer oxygen and provide uterine massage. (6-1.9) (FRASA p. 485)

27.

D. Massage of the mother's uterus is provided to control excessive bleeding that may occur following delivery. Uterine massage helps to stimulate contractions, which causes the uterus to regain muscle tone and reduce uterine size. This will reduce bleeding. (6-1.9) (FR7 p. 440; FRASA p. 485)

28.

C. In multiple births (twins, triplets) the infants may share a placenta or have separate ones. (6-1.1) (FRASA p. 488)

29.

D. In multiple births, about 33 percent of all the deliveries of the second infant are breech. A breech delivery is one in which the fetal buttocks or the lower extremities are the first to present in the birth canal. (6-1.6) (FRASA p. 488)

30.

C. Ensuring the adequacy of the airway, breathing, and circulation always is a priority treatment for all patients. Oxygen administration is the next priority, followed by managing bleeding from the vagina. Transport is the last step. (*) (FR7 p. 449; FRASA p. 379)

31.

C. The pregnant trauma patient is able to compensate for blood loss because of an overall increase in body fluid. Late-pregnancy patients are at greater risk for injuries to the uterus, liver, and spleen or rupture of the mother's diaphragm, even at relatively low speeds. Potential fetal injuries may occur as well. The mother was unrestrained and the potential for injury is present. The best answer presented is to recognize the compensatory capability of the pregnant patient. Encourage the patient to seek medical care and attention. (6-1.4) (FR7 p. 447; FRASA p. 335)

32.

D. Determining if any over-the-counter medications are taken is an appropriate question—but not as important as determining the pain characteristics. Evaluation of the quality of the pain will allow you to determine if the patient is experiencing labor pains or pain related to the accident. (6-1.4) (FR7 pp. 426–427; FRASA p. 480)

33.

C. This patient should be evaluated for signs of crowning. The signs and symptoms presented may indicate immediate delivery. If the patient is crowning, prepare for delivery. (6-1.3) (FR7 pp. 423–424; FRASA pp. 479–480)

34.

C. You should suction the mouth and nose of the infant as soon as the head is delivered and prior to delivery of the rest of the body. After the torso is delivered, the newborn may breathe deeply due to the chest not being constricted in the birth canal. Suctioning the mouth and nose prior to delivery of the torso will help prevent aspiration of the fluids in the mouth and nose. (6-1.7) (FR7 p. 430; FRASA pp. 482–483)

35.

B. You should suction the mouth prior to suctioning the nose. Suctioning the mouth first will prevent aspiration of fluid. Placing the bulb syringe correctly and then compressing the bulb will force the fluid into the lungs. By advancing the tip of the bulb syringe too deeply into the pharynx, the newborn may become bradycardic (slow heart rate). Suction the mouth and nose before stimulating the newborn to remove all secretions prior to spontaneous breathing. (6-1.7) (FR7 p. 431; FRASA p. 483)

36.

D. The pregnant patient who is near full term may experience hypotensive syndrome when lying on her back. To prevent this condition, place the patient supine with her right hip elevated. (6-1.4) (FR7 p. 448; FRASA p. 480)

37.

D. You should avoid applying pressure to the infant's fontanel. The fontanel is the soft area on the infant's head. Gentle pressure can be applied horizontally to prevent an explosive delivery. (6-1.7) (FR7 p. 428; FRASA p. 482)

38.

A. When the placenta appears, grasp it and gently glide it from the vagina. Under no circumstances should you pull the placenta from the vagina. Do not delay transport while waiting for delivery of the placenta. The placenta must be transported to the hospital with the patient; do not dispose of it. The physician will need to examine it. (6-1.8) (FR7 p. 439; FRASA pp. 484–485)

39.

A. The patient that presents with a limb presentation should be placed in a supine position with the head lower than the rest of her body and the hips elevated. This position will increase the gravity and slow the progress of the fetus through the birth canal. Administer oxygen if possible and prepare the patient for immediate transport upon arrival of the EMS crew. Never push or pull a presenting limb into the vagina. Never try to manipulate the fetus into the correct position by inserting your hand into the vagina. (6-1.6) (FR7 pp. 444–445; FRASA p. 487)

40.

C. The infant born before the 38th week of pregnancy is considered premature. Infants weighing less than $5\frac{1}{2}$ pounds at birth are considered premature. Premature babies appear smaller and skinnier, with red and wrinkled skin. Premature babies usually will have a single crease across the soles of their feet. The premature infant will have fine silky hair and very small breast nodules. The premature infant will not have cartilage in the outer ear. (6-1.10)

41.

B. This infant was born before the 38th week of gestation, which makes the infant premature. Premature infants need special care because their lungs and organs are not fully developed. Premature infants must be kept warm by using warmed blankets or a plastic bubble swaddle. Never forcefully direct oxygen into the premature infant's face; hold the end of the oxygen tubing approximately $\frac{1}{2}$ inch above the infant's mouth and nose. You should suction secretions gently, using the bulb syringe. To prevent heat loss, cover the premature infant's head, leaving the face exposed. (6-1.10) (FR7 p. 446; FRASA p. 488)

42.

B. Place this patient in a supine position with her hips elevated. This position will help to keep the fetus from putting pressure on the cord. All of the other positions listed may increase pressure on the cord. (6-1.4) (FR7 p. 445; FRASA p. 487)

43.

A. You should place your gloved hand into the vagina and gently push the presenting part of the fetus back and away from the pulsating cord. This is an acceptable time for you to place your gloved hand into the vagina. (6-1.4) (FR7 p. 445; FRASA p. 487)

44.

C. This patient's breathing has become inadequate. You must immediately establish an airway and provide positive pressure ventilation. (6-1.4) (FR7 pp. 100–103; FRASA pp. 103, 487)

INFANTS AND CHILDREN 6-2

45.

D. A neonate refers to the first 4 weeks of life; an infant, up to 12 months; a toddler, from 1–3 years; and a preschooler, from 3–6 years of age. (6-2.1) (FR7 p. 461; FRASA p. 497)

46.

B. A toddler, a child from 1–3 years of age, creates an assessment challenge for the emergency responder. Remain calm and try to distract the child with a toy or other object during the assessment. (6-2.1) (FR7 p. 462; FRASA p. 497)

47.

D. The adolescents (12–18 years old) believe that nothing bad can happen to them and are able to use abstract and concrete thinking skills. They may take risks that lead to trauma. If injured, they fear disfigurement and disability. (6-2.1) (FR7 p. 463; FRASA p. 497)

48.

B. Infants have a faster metabolic rate that uses more oxygen than that of the adult patient. An infant's rib cage is more pliable, resulting in less rib injury but in increased injury to the internal organs. Children proportionally have larger heads, predisposing them to head injuries. A child's skin surface area is large compared to its mass, which can increase a child's exposure to a cold environment, causing hypothermia. (6-2.1) (FR7 pp. 461–465; FRASA p. 501)

49.

D. Children have a smaller circulating blood volume than that of adults. Bleeding must be controlled quickly. A seemingly small blood loss in an adult could be life-threatening to the infant or child. (6-2.1) (FR7 pp. 461–465)

50.

D. Children lack the vocabulary and body awareness that adults possess to accurately describe symptoms and assist with care. The adult is able to separate the emotional aspects of illness or injury. The best answer is the most direct answer, "My left arm hurts just below the elbow." (6-2.2) (FR7 pp. 461–463; FRASA p. 497)

51.

C. The overriding treatment goal for infants and children is to anticipate and recognize respiratory problems. The leading medical cause of cardiac arrest in the infant or child is respiratory failure. Quickly manage and support respiratory compromise in the infant or child patient. (6-2.3) (FR7 p. 471; FRASA pp. 509)

52.

C. Signs of early respiratory distress include intercostal retractions, nasal flaring, and increased respiratory rate. They also may include supraclavicular and subcostal retractions, neck muscle retractions, audible breathing sounds including stridor, wheezing and grunting, and "see-saw" respirations. The infant or child progresses from early respiratory distress (compensated respiratory failure) to decompensated respiratory failure to respiratory arrest. In an infant or child, bradypnea (slow breathing) is a sign of respiratory distress, not early respiratory failure. (6-2.3) (FR7 p. 473; FRASA p. 502)

53.

A. The signs of respiratory arrest include the signs described in the question as well as weak or absent peripheral pulses and hypotension in patients over 3 years of age. Patients presenting with these signs require aggressive ventilatory and airway management. (6-2.3) (FR7 p. 473; FRASA p. 500)

54.

C. In addition to the early signs of respiratory distress (compensated respiratory failure), decreased muscle tone should alert you that your patient is in the advanced stages (decompensated respiratory failure). Neck muscle use, "see-saw" respirations, and nasal flaring are all early signs of respiratory distress (compensated respiratory failure). (6-2.3) (FR7 p. 473; FRASA p. 500)

55.

A. This child patient is presenting with a partial airway obstruction. He is moving air and is pink in color. The treatment for a partial airway obstruction with adequate air movement is to place the patient in a position of comfort, administer oxygen if available, and encourage the patient to remove the obstruction by coughing. (6-2.4) (FR7 p. 114; FRASA pp.138–140)

56.

D. The management of an infant with a complete airway obstruction includes placing the infant in a head-down position during the back blows and chest thrusts. This position makes use of gravity to help move the obstruction from the infant's airway. Abdominal thrusts are contraindicated in infants. (6-2.4) (FR7 p. 115; FRASA pp. 138–140)

57.

A. During suctioning of an infant's or child's airway, oxygen is removed as well as any debris or secretions. For this reason, limit suctions to no longer than 5–10 seconds. (6-2.4) (FRASA p. 127)

58.

A. Infants and children require about 5–10 ml/kg of body weight for each ventilation. (6-2.4)

59.

B. Avoid the use of a nasopharyngeal airway in adults, infants, and children with possible head trauma and mid-face trauma. Moving and maintaining the head in a neutral position and manual airway control with the jaw-thrust technique are appropriate management. (6-2.4) (FR7 p. 128)

60.

B. Early signs of severe shock, or hypoperfusion, in children are uncommon because their blood vessels constrict efficiently, which helps to maintain the blood pressure. When the blood pressure does fall, it drops quickly. Frequently the child or infant may go into cardiac arrest from this rapid drop. When pediatric patients deteriorate because of hypoperfusion, they deteriorate faster and more severely than adults. (6-2.7) (FR7 p. 476; FRASA pp. 508–509)

61.

B. The peripheral pulse is absent or weak in the child with shock (hypoperfusion). An altered mental status, delayed capillary refill, and a rapid respiratory rate are also present. (6-2.7) (FR7 pp. 476–477; FRASA pp. 508–509)

62.

C. The normal temperature of an infant or child is 98° F, or 36.5° C. (*) (FRASA p. 505)

63.

A. Cardiac events in children and infants are uncommon. Common causes of shock (hypoperfusion) include diarrhea, dehydration, vomiting, trauma, blood loss, infection, and abdominal injuries. (6-2.7) (FR7 p. 476; FRASA pp. 508–509)

64.

C. Adequate tissue perfusion in the infant or child patient is characterized by normal capillary refill (less than 2 seconds), pulse rate and strength, warmth and color of the hands and feet, urinary output, and mental status. Alteration of any one of these factors can be an indication of inadequate perfusion. (6-2.7) (FR7 p. 467; FRASA p. 506)

65.

D. A rapid respiratory rate may indicate hypoperfusion in the child patient. A bounding peripheral pulse does not indicate hypoperfusion; blood is being pumped adequately to the extremities. A prolonged capillary refill of less than 2 seconds is normal. (6-2.7) (FR7 pp. 476–477; FRASA pp. 508–509)

66.

D. Causes of seizure activity in children and adults are similar with one notable exception, fever. Febrile seizures are common in children but occur rarely in adults. (6-2.5) (FR7 p. 474; FRASA p. 512)

67.

D. In adults, infants, and children, a seizure that lasts longer than 15 minutes or recurs without a recovery period is called status epilepticus. Ensure an airway, be prepared to suction the airway, and provide positive pressure ventilation. (6-2.6) (FRASA p. 512)

68.

D. Common injury patterns in children who are unrestrained in a vehicle accident include head and neck injuries. This is due to the head size of children and the likely impact with the dashboard. (6-2.7) (FRASA pp. 507–508)

69.

A. The leading cause of death in children is trauma. This includes vehicle accidents, bicycle accidents, ATV accidents, falls, recreational activities, and pedestrian accidents. The primary killer of children is the automobile. (6-2.7) (FR7 p. 481; FRASA pp. 507–508)

70.

A. When providing positive pressure ventilation to the infant or child, the rescuer must take special care to avoid high ventilatory pressure, which can lead to gastric distention. Gastric distention can be avoided or reduced by using cricoid pressure during ventilation. (6-2.4) (FR7 p. 112; FRASA p. 111)

71.

A. Rapid reporting of injuries is not a general indicator of child abuse. Reports of injuries would be delayed. Additional signs of abuse include multiple abrasions, lacerations, bruises, malnourishment, untreated chronic illness, and injuries on both the front and back or both sides of the child's body. (6-2.8) (FR7 pp. 492–493; FRASA p. 513)

72.

D. A child of abuse will commonly be the victim of a combination of all the forms of abuse listed: physical, emotional, and sexual abuse, as well as neglect. (6-2.8) (FR7 p. 490; FRASA p. 513)

73.

A. Only document objective, not subjective, information. Subjective information such as "The patient was abused" must be avoided. Only document objective information statements or observations made. (6-2.9) (FR7 p. 490; FRASA p. 515)

74.

D. Critical-incident stress debriefing for First Responders is frequently required following a traumatic injury to an infant or child. Stress and anxiety are common and stem from a lack of experience in treating children, the fear of failure, and identifying patients with the First Responder's own children. (6-2.10) (FR7 p. 494; FRASA p. 515)

7 EMS Operations

module objectives

Questions in this module relate to D.O.T. objectives 7-1.1 to 7-1.10.

DIRECTIONS Each of the questions or incomplete statements below is followed by suggested answers or completions. Select the **one answer** that is best in each case.

1. When you are driving to an emergency scene, most state laws allow:
    A. exceeding the speed limit without regard for the safety of others.
    B. proceeding through a traffic light without regard for the safety of others.
    C. parking anywhere at any time without any restriction.
    D. exceeding the speed limit while respecting the safety of others.

2. You are responding to a medical emergency. Which of the following actions is considered unsafe while driving the emergency response vehicle?
    A. entering a curve at the outside or high part
    B. accelerating gradually as you leave a curve
    C. driving only as fast as you feel comfortable
    D. braking to the proper speed after entering a curve

3. The use of an escort vehicle is considered dangerous; however, it can be used with extreme caution in which of the following circumstances?
    A. when you are unfamiliar with how to get to the scene
    B. on a four-lane highway
    C. when traffic is congested
    D. when responding through an urban area with intersections

4. Which of the following situations is **true** pertaining to the use of a police escort?
    A. Use escorts only if you cannot quickly travel through high-traffic areas.
    B. Use escorts only at traffic intersections, railroad crossings, and bridges.
    C. Use escorts only if you are unfamiliar with how to get to the scene.
    D. Use escorts to reduce the time it takes you to drive through traffic.

5. You are dispatched to an emergency. Which of the following is considered **essential information** in order to respond to the call?
    A. gender of the patient
    B. age of the patient
    C. name of the patient
    D. location of the patient

6. You are approaching a railroad crossing while responding to the scene of an emergency. The gate is down and you see a long train approaching. You determine the train is traveling very slowly. You should:
    A. shine your spotlight on the train engine to signal the engineer to stop.
    B. cross the tracks quickly with your warning lights on.
    C. wait for the train to pass if there is no immediate alternative route.
    D. proceed through the intersection since the train must stop for an emergency response vehicle.

7. Which of the following statements is **true** regarding emergency vehicle driving techniques?
    A. It is dangerous to brake after entering a curve.
    B. You should accelerate suddenly as you leave a curve.
    C. Stopping distance is shortened when vehicle speed increases.
    D. Brakes in emergency vehicles equipped with antilocking brakes should be pumped.

8. Your patient has vomited on the long spine board. Your first action when cleaning the spine board is to:
   A. spread a germicide on top of the vomitus.
   B. sweep the vomitus into a bag with a broom.
   C. clean up visible vomitus with disposable towels.
   D. sterilize the area with a chemical sterilant.

9. Intermediate-level disinfection should be used for surfaces that come into contact with intact skin. Which solution of household bleach and water should be used for intermediate-level disinfection?
   A. 1:1
   B. 1:10
   C. 1:100
   D. 1:1000

10. To clean emergency equipment that comes in contact with a patient's intact skin, such as a stethoscope, you should:
    A. immerse in an EPA-registered sterilant for 6 to 10 hours.
    B. immerse in an EPA-registered sterilant for 10 to 45 minutes.
    C. use low-level disinfection, 1:100 ratio of bleach and water.
    D. use intermediate-level disinfection, 1:10 ratio of bleach and water.

11. Which of the following best describes the role of the EMS First Responder on a scene where a patient is entrapped within a motor vehicle?
    A. extrication technician
    B. disentanglement worker
    C. patient care provider
    D. scene safety officer

12. After you have determined a vehicle is safe to approach, the most appropriate way to approach your patient trapped in the vehicle is to:
    A. approach from the rear of the patient.
    B. approach directly facing the patient.
    C. approach from the patient's left side.
    D. approach from the patient's right side.

13. When preparing to extricate your patient from a motor vehicle, all of the following are acceptable **except** to:
    A. inform the patient what you are about to do and what to expect.
    B. instruct the patient to focus on an object directly in front of him or her.
    C. have the patient lie across the seat for protection prior to extricating.
    D. look the patient directly in the eyes while speaking to him or her.

14. You have received dispatch information while responding to a call that informs you that the patient is trapped in a vehicle. Your first action should be:
    A. stabilization.
    B. gaining access.
    C. disentanglement.
    D. scene size-up.

15. You are preparing to extricate your patient from a vehicle. The access of choice is usually the:
    A. door.
    B. windshield.
    C. side window.
    D. removed roof.

16. After gaining safe access to a patient who is entangled in a motor vehicle, your first emergency treatment should be:
    A. opening the airway.
    B. determining the mental status.
    C. inserting an oropharyngeal airway.
    D. taking manual stabilization of the spine.

17. You have arrived on a motor vehicle crash scene. The police officer states your patient is entangled and access appears to be "complex." You recognize this to be:

    A. access that takes longer than 20 minutes.

    B. access that requires the use of extrication tools.

    C. access that cannot be performed by the typical EMS First Responder.

    D. access that requires the notification of the police.

18. While waiting for help to arrive on a hazardous materials scene, you should protect bystanders by:

    A. advising them to shut off electronics.

    B. advising them to remain calm.

    C. directing them to keep downhill.

    D. directing them to keep upwind.

19. You are the first to arrive at the scene of a possible hazardous materials spill. Your first action should be to:

    A. ensure there are enough additional equipment and personnel.

    B. approach the scene carefully and identify the hazardous material.

    C. protect yourself by donning a hazardous materials protective suit.

    D. secure the scene and prevent the exposure of rescuers and bystanders.

20. The area of a hazardous materials scene where contamination is actually present and treatment is limited to life-threatening conditions is known as the:

    A. hot zone.

    B. warm zone.

    C. cold zone.

    D. safe zone.

21. The criteria for a multiple casualty incident (MCI) are best described by:

    A. any event that involves mass transit or a large building where people may be.

    B. any event that places excessive demands on EMS personnel and equipment.

    C. any event that typically involves more than three emergency vehicles.

    D. any event that requires police, fire, and EMS to respond simultaneously.

22. You are the senior First Responder and have arrived at the scene of a disaster involving many victims. Your responsibility is to assume:

    A. EMS incident manager until relieved.

    B. staging sector command until relieved.

    C. triage sector command until relieved.

    D. supply sector command until relieved.

23. You are the next senior First Responder who arrives after the first responding vehicle on the scene of a mass casualty incident (MCI). Your immediate role will be:

    A. EMS incident manager.

    B. treatment sector officer.

    C. primary triage officer.

    D. staging sector officer.

24. To protect yourself at a scene of a hazardous materials incident, you should position yourself and others:

    A. downhill and downwind.

    B. downhill and upwind.

    C. uphill and downwind.

    D. uphill and upwind.

25. You are on the scene of a multiple-casualty incident and are assigned as the primary triage sector. You open the airway of an unresponsive victim and find that the patient is not breathing. You should:

    A. move on to the next patient.

    B. provide rescue breaths for 1 minute.

    C. call for assistance and start CPR.

    D. tag the patient "red" as a priority patient.

SCENARIO

Questions 26 and 27 refer to the following scenario:

You and your partner Joshua Adam are cleaning the vehicle as one of your daily chores. The alerting system sounds, "Unit One and Unit Four, respond to a four-vehicle crash on I-95, mile marker 147, southbound lane." You and Joshua quickly respond. While en route, dispatch advises you of two patients who are critically injured. As you turn onto 20th Street, you notice Unit Four just ahead of your unit.

26. Your unit is directly behind Unit Four as you both approach a busy intersection. Which of the following practices should you follow?

A. Use the same siren mode that Unit Four is currently using.

B. Position yourself so motorists can see both units at a glance.

C. Follow Unit Four as closely as possible through the intersection.

D. Follow Unit Four through the intersection without using your siren.

27. You and Joshua Adam have attended to a critically injured trauma patient. Which of the following best describes the correct procedure for cleaning the splinting equipment that has been returned to you and has dried blood on it?

A. Immerse the splint in an EPA-registered sterilant for 10–45 minutes.

B. Immerse the splint in an EPA-registered sterilant for 6–10 hours.

C. Wipe the equipment carefully with a 1:10 solution of bleach and water.

D. Wipe the equipment carefully with a 1:100 solution of bleach and water.

SCENARIO

Questions 28–30 refer to the following scenario:

You and your partner Russ are reviewing your department's protocol when the alerting system sounds: "Unit One, respond to an automobile crash with injuries at 1729 17th Avenue." You both quickly move to the emergency vehicle. While you are en route to the accident scene, dispatch advises you that a bystander stated there are nine persons injured, some of whom are not responding and have bad injuries. You advise dispatch to activate the multiple-casualty incident plan.

28. What criteria did you use to determine that the multiple-casualty incident plan would need to be implemented?

A. This event will likely take longer than 2 hours to complete.

B. This event and location will limit the number of rescuers on the scene.

C. This event will require an emergency response from EMS, fire, and police.

D. This event will place excessive demand on personnel and equipment.

29. Your unit is the first to arrive on the crash scene and you are the most senior First Responder. Your initial role would be:

A. primary triage manager.

B. primary incident manager.

C. primary treatment manager.

D. primary staging manager.

30. Your partner Russ is assigned to the triage sector. Triage is best described as a:

A. system ensuring that ambulances are accessible and transportation occurs with direction of EMS incident manager.

B. system responsible for distributing the medical material and equipment necessary to render care.

C. system that monitors, inventories, and directs available emergency ambulances to the treatment sector.

D. system used for sorting patients to determine the order in which they will receive care and transport.

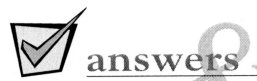

answers & rationales

Following each rationale, you will find a reference to the corresponding D.O.T. objective. A rationale marked with an asterisk denotes material supplemental to the First Responder curriculum. Also included after each rationale are references to where the question topic may be covered in Brady First Responder textbooks. **"FR7" refers to** *First Responder, 7e* (Bergeron, Bizjak, Krause, Le Baudour). **"FRASA" refers to** *First Responder: A Skills Approach, 7e* (Limmer, Karren, Hafen).

1.
D. When operating an emergency response vehicle, you must always respect the safety and well-being of others. This is called due regard for the safety of others. This due regard must be respected when traveling through a traffic light, parking, or exceeding the speed limit. (7-1.2) (FRASA p. 535)

2.
D. Braking to the proper speed after entering a curve is considered dangerous. You should decelerate to a safe speed prior to entering the curve. (7-1.2) (FRASA p. 535)

3.
A. The only acceptable use of an escort vehicle is when the driver of the emergency response vehicle is unfamiliar with how to get to the scene. When using an escort, extreme caution must be exercised because many people pay attention only to the first vehicle. This then puts the second vehicle at risk for a collision. (7-1.2)

4.
C. You should only use a police escort if you are uncertain about how to reach a scene. (7-1.2)

5.
D. The location of the patient is considered essential information needed to respond to a call. Neither the gender nor the age is essential information; however, it is often included as additional information. The name of the patient should not be given over the radio and may be considered a breach of patient confidentiality. (7-1.2) (FR7 p. 502; FRASA p. 534)

6.
C. Never proceed through a crossing gate at a railroad crossing! Simply be calm and wait for the train to pass if there is no immediate alternative route. Trains typically take a very long distance to stop; thus, they are not required to stop for emergency vehicles. (7-1.2)

7.
A. After entering a curve, it is dangerous to apply the brakes. Anticipate the curve and apply the brakes prior to entering the curve; accelerate gradually and carefully as you leave the curve. Stopping distances increase as the speed of the vehicle increases. Vehicles equipped with antilocking brakes should not be pumped; apply the brakes firmly and steadily. (7-1.2) (FRASA p. 535)

8.
C. When cleaning any body fluid or substances that have spilled, you should first protect yourself by wearing gloves, a mask, and eyewear. The visible spill should first be cleaned by using disposable towels to pick up most of the spill. After the spill has been picked up and disposed of properly, you will need to clean the surface with a germicide or mixture of bleach and water. Never try to pick up a spill with a broom, this will only create a larger spill and may cause further contamination. (7-1.2)

9.
B. A ratio of 1:10 or 1 part household bleach and 10 parts water is the correct mixture to use for an intermediate-level disinfection. A 1:1 mixture is too strong; a 1:100 ratio is too weak for an intermediate-level disinfection. A mixture of 1:100 is used for a low-level disinfection such as routine cleaning of the ambulance. A 1:1000 mixture is too weak. (7-1.2)

10.

D. When cleaning equipment that comes in contact with the patient's intact skin, use a 1:10 ratio of bleach and water. A ratio of 1:100 is used for routine housekeeping on surfaces such as floors. Equipment that comes in contact with a patient's mucous membranes should be soaked for 10–45 minutes in an EPA-registered sterilant. Immersion in an EPA-registered sterilant for 6–10 hours is used on equipment that is used invasively, primarily in the hospital. (7-1.2)

11.

C. Your primary role as an EMS First Responder on a crash scene is as a patient care provider. Although you will work closely with the disentanglement team and help to ensure minimal risk to the patient's condition, you will provide emergency care to the patient. (7-1.3) (FR7 p. 503; FRASA p. 590)

12.

B. When approaching a patient inside a vehicle, you should approach directly facing the patient. Approaching the patient from his or her front will help to keep the patient's attention forward, thus keeping the patient from turning his or her head. When you have made direct eye contact with your patient, instruct the patient not to move his or her head. Approaching from the right, left, and behind may cause the patient to move his or her head, possibly further injuring the patient. (7-1.4)

13.

C. Having the patient lie across the seat may further injure the patient. You must maintain in-line spinal stabilization during extrication. It is important to explain to your patient what to expect; this will lessen the patient's apprehension during the extrication process. Having the patient focus on an object directly in front of him or her will help to keep the head and spine in line and not moving. When speaking to your patient, look the patient directly in the eyes; this will help keep the patient from moving his or her head unnecessarily. (7-1.3) (FRASA p. 591)

14.

D. You first must size up the scene. You must determine first that the scene is safe for you to enter. In addition, it will help you organize your resources and prepare for the extrication. A good scene size-up can help reduce injury to the rescuers and patient. (7-1.4) (FR7 p. 499; FRASA p. 586)

15.

A. The door is usually the best access when extricating a patient from a motor vehicle because of its large opening. In addition, it is fairly easy to open. The windshield can be a difficult choice through which to gain access. The side window is usually too small and may cause the spine to be manipulated. The latter routes are referred to as "simple access." The removal of the roof opens the vehicle considerably and can make extrication much easier. Roof removal usually requires special training and equipment and can be costly to the vehicle owner. This route would be an example of "complex access." (7-1.5) (FR7 p. 506; FRASA p. 588)

16.

D. After gaining safe access to your patient, you will stabilize the cervical spine with manual in-line stabilization. Provide the same care as you would on other trauma patients. (7-1.3) (FR7 p. 511; FRASA p. 588)

17.

B. Complex access requires the use of tools or specialized equipment. Access that does not require tools or specialized equipment is known as "simple access." (7-1.5) (FR7 p. 506; FRASA p. 588)

18.

D. While waiting for help to arrive on a hazardous materials incident, you should protect yourself and bystanders by remaining upwind, uphill, and away from the scene. Turning off electronics will not protect you from hazardous materials. (7-1.7) (FR7 p. 516; FRASA p. 549)

19.

D. As the first responding crew on the scene of a hazardous materials incident, you should first secure the scene. Securing the scene will limit the exposure of other rescuers and bystanders. (7-1.6) (FR7 p. 516; FRASA p. 549)

20.

A. The "hot zone" is where contamination is actually present. Treatment in this area is provided by trained personnel wearing protective equipment. Treatment is limited to life-threatening conditions. The "warm zone" is the area outside the hot zone where patients and personnel must remain until they are fully decontaminated. The "cold (or safe) zone" is outside the warm zone. This area is where personnel can remove protective clothing; all life-threatening conditions should have been attended to before the patient reaches this zone. (7-1.7) (FR7 p. 516; FRASA pp. 550–551)

21.

B. An MCI is typically defined as any event that places excessive demands on personnel and equipment. This demand is specific for your individual system. Often an incident involving mass transit or a large building may turn into an MCI; however, the incident must meet the above criteria. A rural system may be taxed by a response of three emergency vehicles; another system may not be taxed by the same response. Often many systems routinely require police, fire, and EMS to respond simultaneously. (7-1.8) (FR7 p. 526; FRASA p. 556)

22.

A. The senior EMS responder who arrives at the scene of a disaster first assumes EMS incident manager until relieved by the predesignated officer. The first person on the scene when multiple casualties are present must assume control of the scene and prepare for the appropriate resources to respond. (7-1.9) (FR7 p. 527; FRASA p. 557)

23.

C. Your immediate role as the next senior First Responder on an MCI is as the primary triage officer. You will remain at this post until relieved by the EMS incident commander. (7-1.9) (FR7 p. 528; FRASA p. 557)

24.

D. To protect yourself and others from possible exposure to a hazardous material, you should position yourself and others uphill and upwind. Positioning in this manner limits exposure for the following reasons: many chemicals being carried with the wind, liquids flowing downhill, and some gases being heavier than air. (7-1.7) (FR7 p. 516; FRASA p. 549)

25.

A. It may be difficult to do, but you must move on to the next patient if you find that there is no breathing or no pulse. Remember you must move on. Attending to this patient would take too many of your much-needed resources. (7-1.10) (FR7 p. 529; FRASA pp. 559–560)

26.

B. You should position your vehicle at a safe distance behind Unit Four but close enough so that motorists can see both units at a glance. Do not follow too closely because reaction time decreases and motorists may think there is only one emergency vehicle and proceed, striking your vehicle. Always use all of your lights and your siren when approaching and proceeding through an intersection. When following another emergency vehicle, use a different siren mode than the other vehicle. (7-1.1) (FRASA p. 537)

27.

C. Clean the equipment with a 1:10 bleach and water solution. (7-1.2)

28.

D. This event will likely place an excessive demand on your personnel and equipment resources. It is far better to activate the MCI plan and have too many rescuers and equipment en route to the scene than to have too few responding. (7-1.8) (FR7 p. 526; FRASA p. 556)

29.

B. If you are the most senior First Responder to arrive on the scene of a multiple casualty incident, your initial role will be that of the EMS incident manager. You will remain the EMS incident manager until relieved by the predesignated officer if there is one. (7-1.9) (FR7 p. 528; FRASA pp. 557–558)

30.

D. Triage is a system that sorts patients to determine the order in which they will receive care and transportation to the hospital. Triage usually divides patients into groups that are high priority, second priority, and lowest priority. (7-1.10) (FR7 p. 528; FRASA p. 559)

Comprehensive
Self-Assessment Exam

DIRECTIONS Each of the questions or incomplete statements below is followed by suggested answers or completions. Select the **one answer** that is best in each case.

1. An example of an unsafe on-scene activity is:
   A. wearing reflective clothing at night.
   B. using latex gloves.
   C. wearing protective clothing.
   D. entering a crime scene quickly.

2. Which of the following is a behavioral response to stress?
   A. depression
   B. overeating
   C. defensiveness
   D. mood swings

3. The single most important way to prevent the spread of infection is by:
   A. wearing latex gloves.
   B. wearing a disposable face mask.
   C. using antiseptic wipes.
   D. vigorous hand washing.

4. You are responding to a possible crime scene. The patient is reported to be bleeding heavily. You should:
   A. make patient contact and immediately begin your treatment.
   B. get access to the residence and speak to the patient from a distance.
   C. wait for police to secure the scene before entering the scene.
   D. position your vehicle on-scene and wait for police to arrive.

5. A patient who nods his head when asked by you if you can assess and treat his injuries has given what type of consent?
   A. implied
   B. minor's
   C. expressed
   D. emancipated

6. The term that means "on both sides" is:
   A. unilateral.
   B. lateral.
   C. bilateral.
   D. proximal.

7. You arrive on the scene and find the patient lying face down. You would record the patient was found in a _____ position?
   A. supine
   B. lateral
   C. prone
   D. Fowler's

8. Which of the following patients is breathing **adequately?**
   A. 6-month-old using his abdominal muscles to breathe at 30 times per minute
   B. 42-year-old breathing irregularly with deep sighs at 8 times per minute
   C. 8-year-old excessively using his neck muscles to breathe at 20 times per minute
   D. 60-year-old breathing with unequal chest expansion at 42 times per minute

9. You are treating an 8-year-old patient who was kicked in the head by a horse. You should open the airway using which of the following maneuvers?
   A. jaw-thrust
   B. head-tilt, chin-lift
   C. hyperextension
   D. head-tilt, flex neck

10. Stimulation of the back of the throat while suctioning a patient may result in:
    A. tachypnea.
    B. bronchospasm.
    C. bradypnea.
    D. bradycardia.

11. When you are preparing to suction the nasopharynx with a French catheter, the length is determined by:
    A. measuring from the tip of the patient's nose to the angle of the jaw.
    B. measuring from the corner of the patient's mouth to the tip of the ear.
    C. measuring from the tip of the patient's nose to the tip of the ear.
    D. measuring from the corner of the patient's mouth to the angle of the jaw.

12. After inserting an oropharyngeal airway, the patient begins to gag. You should:
    A. insert a nasopharyngeal airway in addition to the oropharyngeal airway.
    B. immediately remove the oropharyngeal airway and prepare to suction.
    C. reassure the patient that the oropharyngeal airway is necessary.
    D. do nothing; the gagging will subside within a few minutes.

13. You have determined that the number of patients at the scene has exceeded your ability to effectively manage the situation. You have summoned additional resources. Your next action should be to:
    A. move all patients to the transport area.
    B. immediately begin treating the patients.
    C. perform a focused history on the patients.
    D. begin to triage and prioritize the patients.

14. A deeply unresponsive patient:
    A. may have an intact gag reflex.
    B. responds to tactile stimulation.
    C. may cough when an airway adjunct is placed.
    D. does not respond to pain.

15. Which upper respiratory sound may indicate a liquid substance in the airway?
    A. crowing
    B. snoring
    C. gurgling
    D. stridor

16. While assessing a patient, you find that the patient's skin is pale, cool, and moist. Which of the following would most likely cause this assessment finding?
    A. hyperthermia
    B. hypoperfusion
    C. fever
    D. dehydration

17. All of the following are examples of life threats that should be managed in the initial assessment **except:**
    A. inadequate breathing.
    B. open chest injury.
    C. closed humerus fracture.
    D. major bleeding.

18. When performing a rapid head-to-toe First Responder physical exam on a trauma patient, you are most concerned with:
    A. doing a detailed assessment for each injury site.
    B. obtaining completely accurate vital signs.
    C. obtaining the SAMPLE history.
    D. identifying life-threatening injuries.

19. You arrive on the scene and find a 26-year-old male patient lying supine on the road after falling off his motorcycle. Upon your arrival, he is complaining of severe pain to his pelvis and upper left leg. At this point, you should assume:
    A. he responds to painful stimuli and his oxygen level is adequate.
    B. his pulse is present and his perfusion status is adequate.
    C. he is alert, his airway is open, and he is breathing adequately.
    D. he is alert and he has no internal bleeding or shock.

20. In the medical patient, which of the following provides the most helpful information?
    A. the patient's blood pressure
    B. SAMPLE history
    C. the patient's respiratory status
    D. the patient's pulse rate

21. During the SAMPLE history for a responsive medical patient, the OPQRST question you used to have the patient rate his or her pain on a scale of 1 to 10 is known as:
    A. radiation.
    B. quality.
    C. severity.
    D. provocation.

22. You are assessing a patient who complains of pelvis pain after a fall from a ladder. In your assessment of the pelvis, you should:
    A. not palpate the pelvis, but just visually inspect it.
    B. rock the pelvis, checking for instability.
    C. compress the pelvis inward and downward.
    D. apply firm pressure to the pubic bone.

23. Which of the following would **not** be considered a symptom?
    A. nausea
    B. pain
    C. stridor
    D. lightheadedness

24. Which of the following is the preferred pulse to assess in a 6-month-old patient?
    A. brachial
    B. radial
    C. carotid
    D. femoral

25. The dorsalis pedis pulse is located:
    A. behind the inner ankle bone.
    B. at the bend of the elbow.
    C. behind the knee.
    D. on the top surface of the foot.

26. The first step in the ongoing assessment is to:
    A. check your interventions.
    B. repeat the focused assessment for other injuries or complaints.
    C. reassess and record vital signs.
    D. repeat the initial assessment.

27. You note a change in the patient's mental status after completing your assessment and while you wait for the EMS crew. You should immediately:
    A. take a complete set of vital signs.
    B. assess effectiveness of emergency care.
    C. increase the oxygenation of the patient.
    D. repeat the initial assessment.

28. Which of the following signs found during the ongoing assessment of an adult would indicate the patient's condition is improving?
    A. The patient's breathing was 10 per minute and is now 32 per minute.
    B. The patient's skin color changes from cyanotic to blue-gray.
    C. The patient begins to use his neck muscles and chest accessory muscles to breathe.
    D. The patient's heart rate increases from 32 to 100 bpm.

29. The ongoing assessment should be repeated every _____ minutes in the unstable patient.
    A. 2
    B. 3
    C. 4
    D. 5

30. When you are dealing with a patient who seems hostile or aggressive, it may be necessary to assert your authority. Which position is likely to convey authority?
    A. keeping your eye level below the patient's
    B. keeping your eye level above the patient's
    C. communicating without making eye contact
    D. communicating while staring at the patient

31. The patient you are treating has refused to allow you to assess and treat him. You have determined that the patient was alert and able to make a rational decision. You have made numerous attempts to persuade the patient to be assessed and treated and the patient continues to refuse both. The patient also refuses to sign the refusal-of-care form. You should:
    A. force the patient to sign the form by refusing to leave until it is signed.
    B. have a family member sign the form verifying that the patient refused to sign.
    C. leave the scene without the signature and advise dispatch of the situation.
    D. sign the patient's name for the patient and document the unusual circumstances.

32. Which of the following is **not** a sign of breathing difficulty?
    A. restlessness and agitation
    B. acute abdominal pain
    C. neck and upper chest accessory muscle use
    D. speech broken by a gasp after every few words

33. When providing emergency care for the adult patient with breathing difficulty, you should:
    A. take time to determine the exact cause of the patient's distress.
    B. expose and inspect the chest if trauma was possibly involved.
    C. only provide positive pressure ventilation if the respiratory rate drops below 12 per minute.
    D. consider the patient a low treatment priority.

34. On palpation of the abdomen, you note the abdominal wall is rigid. This is an indication:
    A. that the patient has no abdominal injury.
    B. of an injury to the lungs leading to respiratory distress.
    C. that the femur has potentially been fractured and is bleeding.
    D. of bleeding occurring within the abdomen.

35. The L in the mnemonic SAMPLE stands for:
    A. last time the patient has the symptom.
    B. last oral intake.
    C. lacerations.
    D. length of signs and symptoms.

36. During your initial assessment of a patient who was complaining of difficulty breathing prior to your arrival, you find vomit in the airway; the respiratory rate is 21 per minute with minimal chest rise and a heart rate of 124 bpm. You should immediately:
    A. suction the airway, insert an oropharyngeal airway, and begin pocket-mask ventilation.
    B. suction the airway, apply high-flow oxygen, and continue your assessment.
    C. assess the skin color, temperature, and condition and suction the airway.
    D. insert an oropharyngeal airway and begin bag-valve-mask ventilation.

37. You are treating a patient with an altered mental status who has a respiratory rate of 8 per minute with full, deep breaths. His heart rate is 98 bpm, and his skin is pale, cool and clammy. You should immediately:
    A. begin to provide positive pressure ventilation.
    B. perform a head-to-toe physical exam.
    C. provide oxygen by a nonrebreather mask at 15 lpm.
    D. position the patient in a lateral recumbent position.

38. The hand-off report should contain all of the following information **except:**
    A. chief complaint.
    B. patient medications.
    C. patient diagnosis.
    D. physical exam findings.

39. Exposure to cool night air will frequently reduce a child's distress associated with:
    A. epiglottis.
    B. croup.
    C. asthma.
    D. pulmonary embolism.

40. A common cause of mechanical AED failure is:
    A. cable breakage.
    B. 80-cycle interference.
    C. battery failure.
    D. cold temperature.

41. Which of the following is the primary priority in providing care for a patient in cardiac arrest?
    A. placement of an oropharyngeal airway
    B. administering positive pressure ventilation
    C. obtaining a patient history
    D. attaching the automated external defibrillator

42. The ratio of compressions to ventilations for a 10-year-old is _____ compressions to _____ ventilations.
    A. 30, 2
    B. 15, 1
    C. 5, 1
    D. 5, 2

43. You have encountered a 6-month-old patient who is alert, thrashing about, but not breathing. The mother states the patient was eating a hot dog piece and began to cough and choke. You would immediately:
    A. perform finger sweep in an attempt to remove the obstruction.
    B. begin positive pressure ventilation.
    C. provide five back slaps and five chest thrusts.
    D. perform five to ten abdominal thrusts.

44. The proper depth of compression for a 3-year-old child is:
    A. one-third to one-half the depth of the chest
    B. one-half to three-fourths the depth of the chest.
    C. $1\frac{1}{2}$ inches to 2 inches
    D. 2 to $2\frac{1}{2}$ inches

45. The number one killer in America today is:
    A. automobile accidents.
    B. falls.
    C. cancer.
    D. heart disease.

46. A common finding in women who are having a heart attack is that they:
    A. do not typically have chest pain.
    B. complain of a very severe onset of chest pain.
    C. do not complain of shortness of breath.
    D. complain of sharp pain between their shoulder blades.

47. You are preparing to administer a defibrillation shock using an AED. You notice the patient has a nitroglycerin patch on. You should:
    A. place the adhesive defibrillation pad over the nitroglycerin patch and shock.
    B. not remove the patch, place the defibrillation pad next to the patch, and shock.
    C. remove the patch and wipe the area after you deliver three stacked shocks.
    D. remove the patch and wipe the area with a cloth before defibrillating.

48. An AED should **not** be applied to a patient who is:
    A. less than 1 year of age.
    B. less than 16 years of age.
    C. older than 80 years of age.
    D. more than 200 pounds.

49. You have successfully defibrillated the patient. The patient has a strong radial pulse; however, the breathing is shallow and slow. You should:
    A. wait a few minutes for the respiratory drive to return.
    B. provide oxygen by nasal cannula at 6 lpm.
    C. administer oxygen by nonrebreather mask at 15 lpm.
    D. immediately begin positive pressure ventilation.

50. You have successfully resuscitated your patient after five defibrillations. You should:

 A. leave the AED on and in place and continue with your assessment and emergency care.

 B. remove the AED but leave the electrode pads in place in case the patient arrests again.

 C. completely remove the AED and do not reattach it if the patient goes back into cardiac arrest.

 D. leave the AED in place, turn the AED off, and only turn it on again if the patient stops breathing.

51. The most common cause of an automated external defibrillator (AED) failure is:

 A. battery failure.

 B. lack of training.

 C. cable failure.

 D. outdated pads.

52. The condition in which there is a lack of insulin and a high level of sugar in the blood is called:

 A. hypoglycemia.

 B. insulin shock.

 C. hypoinsulin.

 D. hyperglycemia.

53. In which position should you place a patient with an altered mental status?

 A. supine or prone

 B. semi-Fowler

 C. Trendelenburg

 D. recovery or coma

54. Which symptom is a late sign of stroke?

 A. double vision

 B. stiff neck

 C. headache

 D. garbled speech

55. The stage of a seizure known as the recovery phase, in which the patient's mental status progressively improves over time, is known as the:

 A. aura period.

 B. tonic phase.

 C. clonic phase.

 D. postictal state.

56. The first priority in managing the actively seizing patient who has a known seizure disorder is to:

 A. insert an oropharyngeal airway and begin positive pressure ventilation.

 B. place the patient in a position so that he will not cause further harm to himself.

 C. begin positive pressure ventilation and chest compressions.

 D. perform a head-to-toe physical exam and SAMPLE history.

57. Any seizure that lasts longer than _____ minutes is considered to be a major emergency.

 A. 5

 B. 10

 C. 20

 D. 30

58. A major risk factor for a stroke is:

 A. recent exercise.

 B. fever.

 C. high blood pressure.

 D. seizure.

59. A condition in which the patient has a sudden and temporary loss of consciousness is called:

 A. neuropoxia.

 B. syncope.

 C. postictal.

 D. eclampsia.

60. Which pair of signs and symptoms is the most likely indicator of a severe allergic reaction:

    A. headache and restlessness

    B. respiratory distress and signs of shock

    C. runny or watery eyes

    D. general weakness and abdominal cramping

SCENARIO

Questions 61 and 62 refer to the following scenario:

You arrive on the scene and find a 23-year-old female patient who is in obvious respiratory distress. She has hives covering her face and neck, her skin is red, and you hear stridor with each inhalation. Her respiratory rate is 42 breaths per minute and shallow. Her radial pulse is barely palpable. Her heart rate is 138 bpm.

61. Your first immediate action is to:

    A. begin positive pressure ventilation.

    B. administer oxygen by a nonrebreather mask.

    C. insert a nasopharyngeal airway.

    D. place the patient in the recovery position.

62. The stridor is an indication of:

    A. constriction of the bronchioles.

    B. low blood pressure.

    C. upper airway swelling.

    D. collapse of the lung tissue.

63. A drug of choice in management of the severe allergic reaction is:

    A. epinephrine.

    B. aspirin.

    C. oral glucose.

    D. ipecac.

64. Activated charcoal is the medication of choice for many ingested poisons because it:

    A. inhibits poisons from being absorbed into the body.

    B. neutralizes poisons while in the stomach and GI tract.

    C. prevents poisons from entering the cells by neutralization.

    D. acts as an antidote to most household and commercial poisons.

65. In which position should you place the patient complaining of severe abdominal pain who also presents with signs and symptoms of shock?

    A. left lateral recumbent

    B. supine with feet elevated

    C. semi-Fowler with knees bent

    D. position of comfort for the patient

66. Which of the following persons would likely tolerate a cold environment best and have a reduced risk of hypothermia?

    A. a 3-year-old who is wet from a rain shower

    B. a 20-year-old who has been drinking alcohol

    C. a 34-year-old walking briskly in a stiff wind

    D. a 50-year-old who takes blood pressure medication

67. You are treating a patient who has been bitten by a rattlesnake. Which of the following treatments is correct?

    A. Wash the area around the bite with mild soap and water.

    B. Elevate the injection site above the level of the patient's heart.

    C. Make two small lacerations over the bite and evacuate the wound.

    D. Place a tourniquet superior and inferior to the bite injection site.

68. Choose the phrase that best describes reasonable force to restrain a patient.

    A. use of moderate force to control a dangerous patient whom you have determined a risk

    B. the amount of force needed to overpower and restrain an unruly patient who may injure others

    C. the use of physical and tactile force to subdue a patient and prevent injury to all concerned

    D. minimal amount of force required to keep the patient from injuring self or others

69. The patient who is near full-term pregnancy should be placed in what position?

    A. face down

    B. face up

    C. supine with feet elevated

    D. face up with the right hip elevated

70. Which statement pertaining to the normal delivery of an infant is **correct?**

    A. The placenta most often is delivered 1 to 2 hours after birth.

    B. Gentle pressure should be applied to the fontanel (soft spot) during delivery.

    C. Bleeding after delivery may be up to 1000 cc and is well tolerated.

    D. The placenta must be transported to the hospital for examination.

71. You have just delivered a baby at the scene while you are waiting for the EMS crew. Which of the following is correct pertaining to treatment of this patient?

    A. If the placenta is not delivered within 10 minutes, you should apply traction on the cord to facilitate the delivery.

    B. Assess the mother and newborn, and prepare for the delivery of the placenta within 10 to 20 minutes.

    C. Delay any further treatment until the placenta is completely delivered.

    D. Pack the vagina to prevent post-delivery hemorrhage from occurring.

72. You and your partner have just delivered a baby. The umbilical cord should be cut:

    A. as soon after delivery as possible.

    B. after the cord pulsations cease.

    C. 1 minute after the delivery.

    D. 5 minutes after the delivery.

73. During delivery, the gloved fingertips are positioned on the bony part of the infant's head to:

    A. delay delivery until arrival at the hospital.

    B. prevent an explosive delivery of the head.

    C. stop the delivery until arrival of the EMS crew.

    D. monitor the infant's pulse rate during labor.

74. Your patient has a deep laceration to the upper arm with bright red blood spurting from the wound. Which vessel is likely severed?

    A. brachial artery

    B. femoral artery

    C. cephalic vein

    D. peroneal vein

75. Your patient has been involved in an industrial accident and has a steady flow of dark red blood coming from the leg around the thigh. You should control this patient's bleeding:

    A. during the First Responder physical exam.

    B. during ongoing assessment exam.

    C. during the initial assessment.

    D. after assessing the patient's circulation status.

76. Which order is correct for treating a closed soft-tissue injury?
    A. assure airway and breathing, splint injuries, BSI precautions, treat shock
    B. assure airway and breathing, BSI precautions, splint injuries, treat shock
    C. BSI precautions, assure airway and breathing, treat shock, splint injuries
    D. BSI precautions, treat shock, assure airway and breathing, splint injuries

77. While removing a patient's burned clothing, you find that a portion of the burned shirt has adhered to the patient's skin. You should:
    A. gently remove clothing from the adhered area by pulling it.
    B. cut the shirt around the burned clothing that is adhered to the skin.
    C. apply a burn ointment to the skin with the adhered clothing.
    D. soak the adhered clothing with water, and then remove it.

78. Which of the following is an inappropriate treatment for a patient suffering from burns?
    A. Cover the patient to prevent body heat loss.
    B. Separate burned fingers with sterile dressings.
    C. Stop the burning process by applying water.
    D. Attempt to drain blisters by direct pressure.

79. Which of the following is correct pertaining to the use of a bandage?
    A. A bandage holds a dressing in place.
    B. A bandage must be sterile or free from any organisms.
    C. A bandage must be applied completely around the injured chest.
    D. A bandage usually directly covers an open wound and prevents infection.

80. Blood has soaked through the pressure dressing you applied to your patient's injury. Your next immediate action should be to:
    A. apply a loose tourniquet until you can feel a pulse.
    B. apply a tight tourniquet because the bleeding is uncontrollable.
    C. remove the original dressings and then apply new ones.
    D. apply additional direct pressure to the injury.

81. Leaving the fingertips or toes exposed after bandaging an extremity:
    A. provides for patient comfort through temperature control.
    B. eliminates the potential for circulatory obstruction.
    C. allows for rapid removal of bandages if required.
    D. allows for the assessment of distal circulation.

82. Your patient has a knife embedded in the right side of his chest. Your immediate emergency medical care for this injury should be to:
    A. expose the wound area.
    B. control wound bleeding.
    C. gently remove the object.
    D. manually secure the object.

83. The anterior bone of the lower leg is called the:
    A. fibula.
    B. ulna.
    C. tibia.
    D. femur.

84. Which of the following is an **appropriate** treatment for a patient with a swollen, deformed extremity (fracture)?
    A. Make three attempts to align a fracture if the distal pulses are absent.
    B. Pad the splint to prevent pressure and discomfort to the patient.
    C. To prevent loss of any jewelry around the injury site, leave it in place.
    D. To reduce infection, you should return protruding bones back beneath the skin.

85. When assessing your patient for a potential spine injury, which of the following would you do?
   A. Ask the patient to move to determine the specific area of injury.
   B. Deep palpation near the spine to determine if an injury has occurred.
   C. Flex the patient's neck to assess for a pain response.
   D. Assess the motor and sensory functions in all four extremities.

86. You should leave a full-faced motorcycle helmet in place if:
   A. you suspect airway compromise.
   B. there is vomitus present in the airway.
   C. it is loose and allows for possible swelling of the injured head.
   D. the airway and breathing are adequate and the helmet is firmly holding the head.

87. When providing care for chemical burns to the eye, you should:
   A. delay flushing of the eyes until transport has begun.
   B. flush alkali burns with vinegar for at least 10 minutes.
   C. flush the eyes immediately and continue for at least 20 minutes.
   D. never remove soft or hard contact lenses.

88. Which of the following signs or symptoms indicates a pediatric patient is in respiratory failure?
   A. patient is limp and not responding
   B. nasal flaring
   C. chest retractions and neck muscle use
   D. increased respiratory rate

89. Which of the following signs or symptoms is the best indication of hypoperfusion (shock) in the pediatric patient?
   A. noisy respiration
   B. weak or absent peripheral pulse

   C. pink, warm, and dry skin
   D. capillary refill less than 2 seconds

90. When a parent fails to provide sufficient attention to a child, it is called:
   A. abuse.
   B. neglect.
   C. molestation.
   D. violation.

91. When you are navigating a curve while driving the ambulance, which action could be considered dangerous?
   A. entering the curve on the outside
   B. braking prior to entering the curve
   C. decelerating before entering the curve
   D. accelerating while in the curve

92. To protect yourself and the patient during the extrication process from debris such as glass and metal, you should:
   A. direct the hydraulic spreader operator to be careful.
   B. quickly perform a rapid extrication procedure.
   C. cover the patient and yourself with a tarpaulin.
   D. remove your heavy coat and cover the patient.

93. Which of the following best describes simple access to a patient?
   A. access that takes less than 20 minutes
   B. access that does not require the use of tools
   C. access that requires special training
   D. access gained by using a manually forced tool

94. You are approaching a motor vehicle crash site and notice a truck overturned with a plume of yellow gas surrounding the site. Your first action should be to:

    A. cordon off the area and evacuate all bystanders from the area.

    B. approach the site slowly in an attempt to identify the cargo.

    C. approach the site quickly and remove any injured patients.

    D. assist bystanders to an area downhill and downwind of the site.

95. You are the first to arrive on a scene of a mass casualty incident (MCI). What is your initial role as the first First Responder on-scene?

    A. treatment manager

    B. incident manager

    C. triage officer

    D. staging sector

96. You are at the scene of an MCI and have been assigned to the triage sector. Your patient has sustained a large burn. He has an open airway and is breathing adequately. You would prioritize this patient as:

    A. red—high priority.

    B. yellow—second priority.

    C. green—low priority.

    D. black—lowest priority.

SCENARIO

Questions 97 to 100 refer to the following scenario:

You arrive on the scene and find a 32-year-old male patient who was stabbed in the chest following an altercation in a parking lot.

Upon your arrival at the scene, you find the patient lying supine in a large pool of blood. He is fully clothed and his shirt is soaked in blood. His face and neck are cyanotic. He has blood and vomitus coming from the mouth.

97. Your first immediate action is to:

    A. suction the airway.

    B. begin positive pressure ventilation.

    C. expose the patient.

    D. assess the scene to ensure it is safe to enter.

98. Following this action, you would next perform what immediate action?

    A. Suction the airway.

    B. Begin positive pressure ventilation.

    C. Remove the clothing and assess the bleeding.

    D. Insert an oropharyngeal airway.

As you continue with your assessment, you find the airway is clear, and the patient is breathing 42 times per minute with shallow breaths. His radial pulse is weak and rapid. His skin is pale, cool, and clammy.

99. Your next immediate action is to:

    A. insert an oropharyngeal airway.

    B. begin positive pressure ventilation.

    C. perform a First Responder head-to-toe exam.

    D. suction the airway.

100. You expose the patient and note a stab wound to the front of the chest. You should immediately:

    A. call for transport of the patient.

    B. apply a nonrebreather mask to the patient.

    C. begin a head-to-toe exam to inspect for other injuries.

    D. apply a nonporous dressing to the wound, taped on three sides.

Following each rationale, you will find a reference to where the question topic can be found within Brady First Responder textbooks. **"FR7" refers to *First Responder, 7e*** (Bergeron, Bizjak, Krause, Le Baudor). **"FRASA" refers to *First Responder: A Skills Approach, 7e*** (Limmer, Karren, Hafen).

1.

D. An example of an unsafe on-scene activity is entering a crime scene too quickly, before the situation has been controlled by law enforcement. (FR7 p. 48; FRASA p. 24)

2.

B. People react to stress differently. Behavioral reactions include overeating, increased alcohol and drug use, teeth grinding, hyperactivity, or the lack of energy. Choices A, C, and D are all psychological reactions to stress. In addition to behavioral and psychological reactions, some people react socially (increased interpersonal conflicts) or cognitively, which includes confusion and loss of objectivity. (FRASA p. 27)

3.

D. The single most important way to prevent the spread of infection is by hand washing. Contaminants can be removed from the hands by 10 to 15 seconds of vigorous scrubbing with plain soap. (FR7 p. 42; FRASA p. 19)

4.

C. As a First Responder, you will be called to crime scenes or dangerous situations. Never enter a possibly dangerous scene; always position your vehicle away from the scene and wait for the police to stabilize the situation. Parking in view of the scene may endanger you, as well as escalate the anger of the people on the scene due to your not making patient contact. If you enter a scene and it then becomes hostile, quickly leave the scene and wait for the police to arrive and secure it. (FR7 pp. 48, 50; FRASA pp. 24–25)

5.

C. By nodding his head when asked if you can assess and provide treatment, he is giving his expressed consent for medical care. Expressed consent does not have to come in the form of verbal permission.

Implied consent is used if the patient is unresponsive, or if he has an altered mental status or is not able to make a rational decision regarding his care. Minor consent is used for children and adolescents who are typically less than 18 years of age. (FR7 p. 22; FRASA p. 36)

6.

C. The term that means "on both sides" is bilateral. Lateral is toward the side or away from the mid-line. Unilateral means on one side. Proximal means near the point of reference. (FR7 p. 584; FRASA p. 50)

7.

C. A face-down position is referred to as a prone position. Supine describes a patient lying on his back with his face up. Lateral describes a patient on his side. A Fowler's position refers to a patient who is in a seated position with his upper body at a 45-degree angle or greater. (FR7 p. 57; FRASA p. 50)

8.

A. In an infant, the chest muscles are not well developed; therefore, the infant must rely on the abdominal muscles to breathe. Thus, it is normal for a 6-month-old to breathe with the use of his abdominal muscles. Excessive use of the muscles in the neck is a significant indication of respiratory distress. Irregular respiration and deep sighing breathing may be an indication of an injury to the respiratory center. These respiratory patterns do not typically produce an adequate breathing status. Unequal movement of the chest is an indication of a chest wall injury or, potentially, a lung. (FR7 p. 100; FRASA pp. 102–103)

9.

A. Using the jaw-thrust maneuver will open the airway without compromising the spine. Use the jaw-thrust maneuver whenever you suspect the possibility of a spinal injury. The head-tilt, chin-lift maneuver will compromise the spine when opening the airway. (FR7 p. 102; FRASA p. 99)

10.

D. Stimulating the back of the throat while suctioning may result in bradycardia, a slowing of the heart. There are sensitive nerves in this area and, if stimulated, they may cause a decrease in the heart rate, further complicating the patient's condition. Bronchospasm refers to the constriction of the bronchi. Tachypnea is a fast breathing rate. Bradypnea is a slow breathing rate. (FRASA p. 127)

11.

C. The correct method to measure the length of the catheter needed to suction the nasopharynx is from the tip of the patient's nose to the tip of the ear.

12.

B. If the patient begins to gag or vomit after inserting the oropharyngeal airway, you must immediately remove the airway and prepare to suction. Insert a nasopharyngeal airway. The oropharyngeal airway must only be used in the completely unresponsive patient. (FR7 p. 126; FRASA p. 124)

13.

D. You should first triage and prioritize the patients. This will help to organize the emergency care they receive. The critically injured patient should be treated before patients with minor injuries. Triaging will help to organize the whole scene. Treating and transporting patients in an organized manner will reduce on-scene time and increase the rate of survival of the patients. (FR7 p. 528; FRASA p. 560)

14.

D. An unresponsive patient does not respond to any stimuli. This patient typically does not cough or gag when an airway adjunct is placed into the throat. (FR7 p. 154; FRASA p. 217)

15.

C. Liquid substances in the upper airway result in gurgling sounds. Crowing and stridor are produced on inspiration and are associated with upper-airway swelling or muscle spasm. Snoring is caused by a partial airway obstruction of the tongue or epiglottis. (FR7 p. 113; FRASA p. 99)

16.

B. The patient who presents with pale, cool, and moist skin is likely in a state of decreased perfusion (hypoperfusion). This state of hypoperfusion should clue you to look for the onset of shock. Hyperthermia, an elevated body core temperature, usually presents with hot, red skin. (FR7 p. 309; FRASA p. 335)

17.

C. Life threats that require immediate treatment during the initial assessment include airway control, breathing inadequacy, injuries to the chest, and major bleeding. Fracture management is a secondary injury and is not considered a life threat. (FR7 p. 143; FRASA p. 461)

18.

D. When performing the rapid head-to-toe First Responder physical exam on a trauma patient, you are most concerned with identifying life-threatening injuries. (FR7 p. 159; FRASA p. 198)

19.

C. Because the patient is complaining when you arrive on the scene, you could assume he is alert, his airway is open, and he is breathing adequately. If his airway were obstructed or if he were not breathing adequately, he would not be able to complain. You cannot determine the circulation or perfusion status until after you have checked the pulse and skin temperature, color, and condition. (FR7 p. 100; FRASA p. 216)

20.

B. The patient's SAMPLE history will typically provide more information in the medical patient than the physical exam. In the trauma patient, more information is gained from the physical exam. (FR7 p. 165; FRASA p. 227)

21.

C. Severity questions relate to how bad the pain is. Many patients can rate the pain on a scale from 1 to 10 with 10 being the worst. This method will help you when you reevaluate the patient. If the pain was originally a 4 and is now an 8, the pain has become worse. (FRASA p. 252)

22.

A. If a patient complains of pelvis pain or there is obvious injury to the pelvis, do not palpate the pelvis. Palpating or manipulating the pelvis may cause further injury and severe pain. If the patient does *not* complain of pelvis pain or is unresponsive, palpate by placing both hands on the anterior lateral wings of the pelvis. When palpating the pelvis, you should use gentle inward and downward compression. Do not rock the pelvis or apply too much pressure. (FR7 p. 175; FRASA p. 467)

23.

C. A symptom is something that the patient must tell you, such as nausea, lightheadedness, and pain. You cannot see, feel, or hear any of these. A sign is an objective finding. It is something that can be seen, felt, or heard by you. Stridor, a high-pitched sound that is an indication of a partially obstructed airway at the level of the larynx, is heard by the First Responder. (FR7 p. 159; FRASA p. 227)

24.

A. The brachial pulse is assessed in the infant patient (less than 1 year of age). In patients older than 1 year of age, the radial pulse and carotid pulse are palpated. A femoral pulse could be assessed in an infant, child, or adult; however, it is not the preferred pulse to assess. (FR7 p. 187; FRASA pp. 219, 220)

25.

D. The dorsalis pedis pulse is located on the top surface of the foot. The posterior tibial pulse is located behind the inner ankle bone. The brachial pulse is located along the inner surface of the upper arm between the bicep and tricep. The popliteal is located behind the knee. (FR7 p. 175; FRASA p. 202)

26.

D. The first step in the ongoing assessment is to repeat the initial assessment. This is followed by reassessing and recording vital signs, repeating the focused assessment, and rechecking your interventions. (FR7 p. 178; FRASA p. 229)

27.

D. If the patient's condition has worsened, you should first perform an ongoing assessment, which begins with a repeat of the initial assessment. (FR7 p. 143; FRASA p. 229)

28.

D. The patient's heart rate was too slow (bradycardia) and increased to 100 bpm, which is within a normal range in the adult patient. It is not a sign of improvement when the patient who was breathing too slowly (bradypnea) is now breathing too fast (tachypnea). The patient's skin color is a good indication of the effectiveness of oxygenation of the patient. Skin color that changes from cyanotic to blue-gray is a sign of inadequate oxygenation and poor perfusion of the tissue. When a patient begins to use accessory muscles to breathe, the patient is deteriorating and needs to be ventilated with positive pressure ventilation. (FR7 p. 178; FRASA p. 229)

29.

D. The ongoing assessment should be repeated every 5 minutes in the critical patient. Repeat the ongoing every 15 minutes in the stable patient. (FR7 p. 178; FRASA p. 229)

30.

B. Keeping your eye level above a patient's who is hostile or aggressive will help to assert your authority. This simple positioning can make a great deal of difference in the difficult patient. Positioning yourself below the patient's eye level may convey a submissive position. You should avoid staring at a patient; make eye contact just as you would in a normal conversation. Some patients are on the edge of aggression, and using the correct body language can make a difference in the patient's demeanor. (FR7 p. 271; FRASA p. 315)

31.

B. If the patient will not sign the refusal-of-care form, have a family member, police officer, or bystander sign, stating that the patient refused to sign. The family member or police officer is witnessing that the patient refused to sign the document; they are not signing the refusal for the patient. They are witnesses for your protection. The patient may state later that he or she wanted to be treated and did not sign the report. You must ensure that the patient was alert and able to make a rational decision. (FR7 p. 21; FRASA p. 37)

32.

B. Abdominal pain is not a sign of respiratory distress. Restlessness and agitation are signs that the brain is not getting enough oxygen. Accessory muscle use is a sign of inadequate breathing. The muscles of the neck and upper chest and the diaphragm are used to try to force more air into the lungs. It is an indication of respiratory distress when a patient must gasp for air between every few words. This leads to a broken pattern of speech that is easily recognized by the First Responder. (FR7 p. 100; FRASA p. 102)

33.

B. It is not important to determine the cause of a patient's breathing difficulty, except for the trauma patient. Expose and inspect the trauma patient's chest and treat accordingly. You should provide positive pressure ventilation whenever the rate of respiration or the depth of respiration is inadequate. Patients with breathing difficulty are considered priority patients. (FR7 p. 335; FRASA pp. 182–183)

34.

D. A rigid abdominal wall is a sign of irritation occurring in the abdominal cavity from bleeding or some other source. (FR7 pp. 174, 251; FRASA p. 377)

35.

B. The "L" in the SAMPLE history stands for last oral intake. This is asking when the patient last had something to eat or drink. The S stands for signs and symptoms, A for allergies, M for medications, P for past medical history, and E for events prior to the incident. (FR7 p. 165; FRASA p. 228)

36.

A. The airway must first be cleared with suction, followed by insertion of an oropharyngeal airway. Because the patient has a shallow depth of respiration, you must begin positive pressure ventilation by either a pocket mask or bag-valve mask. (FR7 p. 129; FRASA p. 126)

37.

A. You should provide positive pressure ventilation immediately. This patient has an adequate depth (volume) of respiration; however, he has an inadequate respiratory rate. Either an inadequate respiratory rate or an inadequate tidal volume will make the patient's respiratory status inadequate, requiring positive pressure ventilation. (FR7 p. 100; FRASA p. 102)

38.

C. The hand-off report must contain pertinent information to allow for a smooth transition from the First Responder to the EMS crew; however, it would not contain a patient diagnosis. First Responders do not make a patient diagnosis. (FR7 p. 178; FRASA p. 230)

39.

B. Croup, a common childhood condition, is characterized by a high-pitched sound from swelling of the larynx. Exposing the child to the cool night air will frequently diminish the signs and symptoms. (FR7 p. 471; FRASA p. 510)

40.

C. The most common cause of mechanical failure is related to batteries. Ensure that the batteries are properly maintained to prevent this type of equipment failure. (FR7 p. 206; FRASA p. 173)

41.

D. When caring for adult victims of cardiac arrest, defibrillation with the AED should come first over the other actions listed. Delay in rapidly defibrillating the patient can reduce the patient's chances for surviving the cardiac arrest. (FR7 p. 204; FRASA p. 167)

42.

A. The proper compression-to-ventilation ratio for CPR in an adolescent is 30:2. (FR7 p. 194; FRASA p. 163)

43.

C. In an infant who is conscious and choking but not able to move any air, you would immediately perform five back slaps and five chest thrusts and reassess the airway status. If the patient was choking and still able to move air, you would encourage the infant to cough.

44.

A. The proper compression depth for an infant and child is one-third to one-half the depth of the chest. The proper depth of compression in an adult patient is $1\frac{1}{2}$ to 2 inches. Compressions should be deep enough to produce a carotid or femoral pulse with each compression. (FR7 p. 194; FRASA p. 163)

45.

D. Diseases of the heart and blood vessels are the number one killer of people in America today. (FR7 p. 181; FRASA p. 250)

46.

A. A common finding in women who are suffering a heart attack is that they do not have typical type chest pain. Often these women complain of shortness of breath, fatigue, and trouble sleeping. (FRASA p. 253)

47.

D. You should remove nitroglycerin patches and wipe the area with a cloth before defibrillating the patient. If the nitroglycerin patch is not removed, the current from the defibrillator may melt the plastic, causing a fire, or the patch will interfere with effective delivery of the current to the heart. (FR7 p. 206; FRASA p. 171)

48.

A. The AED should not be applied to a patient who is less than 1 year of age. If the patient is less than 8 years of age, it is preferable to use an AED that has pediatric pads to reduce the amount of energy being delivered with each defibrillation. However, if a pediatric pad set is not available, it is recommended that the adult AED be attached to the pediatric patient. (FR7 p. 206; FRASA p. 169)

49.

D. This patient's breathing is shallow and slow, which is inadequate. This inadequate breathing must be assisted by positive pressure ventilation immediately. (FR7 p. 100; FRASA p. 173)

50.

A. After successful resuscitation of the patient, the AED should be left in place and remain on. The AED will continue to assess the patient rhythm and will not deliver a shock unless the rhythm is a shockable rhythm. (FR7 pp. 208–210; FRASA p. 173)

51.

A. Poor maintenance is the most common cause of AED failure. Battery failure causes most failures. Batteries must be maintained on a regular basis. At the beginning of every shift, the AED and batteries should be checked and maintained in good order. (FR7 p. 206; FRASA p. 173)

52.

D. A high level of sugar in the blood is called hyperglycemia. A low blood sugar level in the blood is called hypoglycemia. When insulin production is insufficient, the sugar cannot leave the blood and enter the body cells. This causes an increase in the blood sugar level. (FR7 p. 248; FRASA p. 270)

53.

D. The patient who has an altered mental status should be placed on his or her side. This position will help to protect the patient's airway from vomitus or secretions by allowing the fluid to flow out of the mouth. This position is referred to as the recovery, coma, or lateral recumbent position. (FR7 p. 245; FRASA p. 269)

54.

B. A stiff neck is a late sign of a stroke. There are many different signs and symptoms of neurologic deficit, depending on the location of the brain injury. (FR7 p. 244; FRASA p. 274)

55.

D. The stage of a seizure that is known as the recovery phase is the postictal state. During this period of time the patient's mental status progressively improves. The patient may present with a severe headache or temporary hemiparesis. (FRASA p. 276)

56.

B. Seizures that occur in a patient who has a seizure disorder, commonly epilepsy, are typically self-limited and last only a few minutes. The first priority after ensuring your own safety is to protect the patient from further injury. You would then assess the airway and breathing. (FR7 p. 247; FRASA p. 276)

57.

A. A seizure that last longer than 10 minutes or two or more seizures that occur without a period of consciousness between them is a dire emergency. This condition is referred to as status epilepticus. (FRASA p. 276)

58.

C. A major risk factor for stroke is high blood pressure (hypertension). (FR7 pp. 243–245; FRASA p. 272)

59.

B. Syncope, also known as fainting, occurs when there is a temporary lack of blood and oxygen flow to the brain. It commonly occurs when the patient is standing. When the patient assumes a supine position, the patient improves rapidly.

60.

B. In a severe allergic reaction, the respiratory and circulatory systems are affected. Mild allergic reactions produce hives and itching, whereas a severe reaction would present with respiratory distress and a poor perfusion state, causing signs of shock. (FR7 p. 262; FRASA pp. 338–339)

61.

A. The patient has inadequate breathing and must receive positive pressure ventilation immediately. (FR7 p. 100; FRASA p. 341)

62.

C. Stridor is a sound produced by partial occlusion of the upper airway. In the case of the severe allergic reaction, the upper airway occlusion is due to swelling of the tissue in the larynx. Stridor is typically more prominent on inhalation. (FR7 p. 113; FRASA p. 99)

63.

A. The drug of choice in the treatment of the severe allergic reaction is epinephrine. The properties of the drug cause the bronchioles to dilate and the vessels to constrict, reversing the signs and symptoms of the severe reaction. (FR7 p. 262; FRASA p. 341)

64.

A. Activated charcoal is the medication of choice to use for ingested poisonings. Activated charcoal works by adsorbing the poison and thus inhibiting absorption into the body. (FR7 p. 561; FRASA p. 280)

65.

B. The acute abdomen patient who is in shock (hypoperfusion) should be placed in a supine position with the patient's feet elevated. This position will help to increase perfusion to the brain and other vital organs. (FR7 p. 312; FRASA p. 337)

66.

C. The 34-year-old is middle aged and tolerates cold better than the young and old. This patient is walking briskly, which increases body temperature through muscle contractions. Certain medications and alcohol will decrease a person's ability to tolerate a cold environment. A person who is wet will lose more heat than a dry person. (FR7 p. 266; FRASA p. 289)

67.

A. You should wash the bite area with a mild soap and water, being careful not to aggressively scrub the area. The injection site should be placed slightly lower than the level of the patient's heart. Never lacerate the injection site to try to evacuate the poison; this may further complicate the patient's recovery and does not remove toxins. Tourniquets should not be used in a snake bite injury. Some protocols may use restricting bands; consult your local medical direction. (FR7 pp. 259–260; FRASA pp. 298–299)

68.

D. Simply stated, reasonable force is the minimum amount of force required to keep a patient from injuring self or others. (FR7 pp. 272–273; FRASA p. 316)

69.

D. To prevent supine hypotension syndrome in the patient who is near full term of her pregnancy, place her in a supine position with the right hip elevated or place her on her left side. If placed in a supine position, the weight of the uterus and fetus presses on the inferior vena cava and causes a reduced blood flow to the heart, leading to a decrease in blood pressure. The patient then experiences lightheadedness or faints while lying flat. (FR7 p. 448; FRASA p. 480)

70.

D. The placenta must be transported to the hospital for examination by a physician. The physician will then determine if the delivery was complete. Normal blood loss after delivery is up to 500 cc in the average-sized adult female. The placenta usually delivers within 10 minutes of the fetus and almost always within 20 minutes. Do not apply pressure to the infant's fontanel; this is the soft, depressed area of the infant's head. (FR7 p. 439; FRASA pp. 484–485)

71.

B. The placenta usually delivers within 10 to 20 minutes following delivery. The placenta, enclosed in a plastic bag, should be transported with the patient. This will allow a physician to examine it to confirm that the placenta delivery was complete. Continue to assess the patient while waiting to deliver the placenta. (FR7 p. 439; FRASA p. 484)

72.

B. The umbilical cord should be cut after the pulsations that are present in the cord cease. Two clamps are positioned on the cord prior to cutting the cord. An AP-GAR score is measured in 1 minute and 5 minutes after delivery. (FR7 pp. 437–438; FRASA p. 484)

73.

B. The fingertips of the gloved hand are positioned on the bony part of the infant's head to prevent an explosive delivery. A rapid or explosive delivery can result in tearing of the birth canal. Be sure not to apply pressure to the anterior fontanel, or soft spot. (FR7 p. 439; FRASA p. 482)

74.

A. The brachial artery is located in the upper arm, and arterial bleeding is bright red and spurts with each heart contraction. The femoral artery is located in the upper leg. The cephalic vein is located in the upper arm; however, bleeding from a vein is dark red and steady. The peroneal vein is located in the lower leg. (FR7 p. 355; FRASA p. 58)

75.

C. Severe or major bleeding is identified as bleeding that spurts or has a steady flow of blood. Immediately upon identification, the severe bleeding must be stopped by applying direct pressure. If severe bleeding is identified during the general impression of the initial assessment, you should immediately apply direct pressure to stop the bleeding prior to any other treatment. (FR7 p. 143; FRASA p. 198)

76.

C. When treating a closed soft-tissue injury, you must first take BSI precautions. Next, assure the patient has an open airway and that the patient is breathing adequately. If the patient is not breathing adequately or has a closed airway, stop and correct the airway or breathing problem. After ensuring the airway is adequate, quickly treat for shock. After treating for shock, you should next splint any painful, swollen, or deformed extremities. (FR7 p. 319; FRASA p. 349)

77.

B. You should cut the shirt away from the adhered portion of clothing. Never remove adhered clothing. This can cause extreme pain and further damage the burn site. Never apply ointments of any kind to burns; most often these ointments must be removed at the hospital. (FR7 pp. 342–343; FRASA pp. 389–390)

78.

D. Never attempt to break or drain blisters from a burn; doing so will likely introduce contaminants and increase the possibility of infection. (FR7 pp. 342–343; FRASA p. 390)

79.

A. A bandage holds a dressing in place. A dressing should be sterile and is placed directly on the wound. Common bandages include self-adhering, gauze rolls, and triangular bandages. Even though some bandages are sterile, they do not have to be. (FR7 p. 289; FRASA p. 358)

80.

D. When blood soaks through the original dressings, you should apply direct pressure to the dressing in an attempt to stop the breathing. Tourniquets should only be applied as an absolute last resort. A loose tourniquet will act as a restricting band and cause the pressure in the blood vessel to increase, thus increasing the bleeding. (FR7 p. 289; FRASA p. 330)

81.

D. Leaving the fingertips or toes exposed after bandaging allows for the assessment of circulation. This allows for continuous assessment of the skin color and temperature. Bandages must not impair circulation distal to an injury. (FR7 p. 300; FRASA p. 330)

82.

D. Your first action should be to manually secure the object. This will reduce the likelihood of the object causing further injury or becoming dislodged. Never remove any object that is embedded in the chest. Next, expose the wound site. After exposing the wound site, you should control the bleeding from around the object. Last, use a bulky dressing to help stabilize the object. (FR7 p. 299; FRASA pp. 353–354)

83.

C. The anterior bone of the lower leg is called the tibia. The posterior bone is called the fibula. (FR7 p. 358; FRASA p. 55)

84.

B. Limit your alignment attempt to one if the distal pulse is absent in an extremity. Splints should be appropriately padded to prevent pressure. Any jewelry around the injury site should be removed. **Never** intentionally return broken bone ends to beneath the skin. (FR7 pp. 367–368; FRASA p. 462)

85.

D. You must assess motor (movement) and sensory (feeling) in all the extremities. You should never ask the patient to move in an attempt to determine the anatomical location of a potential spinal injury. This may cause irreversible spinal cord injury. (FR7 p. 402; FRASA p. 442)

86.

D. A helmet should be removed if it interferes with the assessment or management of the airway or breathing. If the helmet does not fit well and excessive head movement occurs within the helmet, it should be removed. It should be left in place if you can properly immobilize the head and the helmet does not allow for head movement. (FR7 p. 407; FRASA p. 449)

87.

C. You must quickly and continuously provide irrigation of the patient's eyes when dealing with eye burns. Do not use any irrigant other than saline or water. Continue flushing the eyes for at least 20 minutes. Remove contact lenses to prevent trapping of chemical agents under the lens. (FR7 p. 345; FRASA p. 393)

88.

A. A patient who is limp and unresponsive is likely suffering from respiratory failure. A patient in respiratory failure needs positive pressure ventilation immediately. Early signs of respiratory distress are nasal flaring, retractions, accessory muscle use, and an increased respiratory rate. (FR7 p. 473; FRASA p. 500)

89.

B. Absent or weak peripheral pulses indicate poor circulation, a sign of hypoperfusion (shock). Other signs are rapid respiratory rate; pale, cool, and clammy skin; decreased mental status; and prolonged capillary refill. (FR7 p. 476; FRASA pp. 508–509)

90.

B. Physical abuse occurs when improper or excessive action is taken so as to injure or cause harm. Neglect is when the caregiver provides insufficient respect or attention to an individual for whom the caregiver is responsible. This may apply to elderly patients or children. (FR7 pp. 487–490; FRASA p. 513)

91.

D. It is dangerous to accelerate while navigating a curve. You should brake or decelerate prior to entering the curve. You should carefully and gradually accelerate after exiting the curve. You should only drive as fast as feels comfortable. You should enter a curve on the outside or highest part. (FRASA p. 536)

92.

C. To protect yourself and the patient from debris, cover up, using a tarpaulin or heavy blanket. Even the most careful spreader operator cannot keep debris from becoming projectiles. A rapid extrication should be performed if the patient's condition requires it or there is a real threat to the well-being of the rescue personnel. Giving your protective clothing to the patient will not protect you. (FR7 p. 511; FRASA p. 591)

93.

B. Simple access is best described as access that does not require the use of tools or specialized equipment. (FR7 p. 506; FRASA p. 588)

94.

A. Your immediate role as First Responder to a possible hazardous material spill is to cordon off the area and evacuate all bystanders. Do not approach the site even if there are patients visible. Move bystanders uphill and upwind. Do not approach the site to try to identify the type of cargo being transported. (FR7 p. 514; FRASA p. 549)

95.

B. Your initial role as the first First Responder on the scene of an MCI is the incident manager. You will remain the incident manager until you are relieved by the designated EMS incident manager. (FR7 pp. 527–528; FRASA p. 556)

96.

B. A patient who has suffered burns but has no airway or breathing problems should be tagged yellow—second priority. Red, the highest priority, is used for airway problems, severe bleeding, and shock. Green is a low priority and is used for patient's suffering from minor burns, minor injuries, and the walking wounded. Black is the lowest priority and is used for the obviously dead patients. (FR7 p. 529; FRASA p. 560)

97.

D. The most important priority is to ensure that the scene is safe for you to enter. Your safety takes precedence over any assessment and treatment. (FR7 p. 143; FRASA p. 180)

98.

A. After ensuring the scene is safe, you must immediately suction the airway to remove the blood and vomitus. (FR7 p. 130; FRASA p. 126)

99.

B. After securing the airway, you must immediately begin positive pressure ventilation. A respiratory rate of 42 per minute and a shallow depth are both indicators of inadequate breathing. (FR7 p. 100; FRASA p. 112)

100.

D. Upon identification of an open wound to the front, side, or back of the chest, you must immediately cover the open wound with a nonporous or occlusive dressing. The dressing should be taped on three sides to allow for air to escape from the wound. A regular dressing is porous and will allow air to continue to enter the chest and may lead to a collapsed lung. The wound must be occluded as quickly as possible to prevent any air from entering the chest. (FR7 pp. 335–336; FRASA p. 353)

Appendix: D.O.T. Objectives

MODULE 1   PREPARATORY

LESSON 1-1   INTRODUCTION TO EMS SYSTEMS

Cognitive Objectives

At the completion of this lesson, the First Responder student will be able to:

1-1.1   Define the components of Emergency Medical Services (EMS) systems.

1-1.2   Differentiate the roles and responsibilities of the First Responder from other out-of-hospital care providers.

1-1.3   Define medical oversight and discuss the First Responder's role in the process.

1-1.4   Discuss the types of medical oversight that may affect the medical care of a First Responder.

1-1.5   State the specific statutes and regulations in your state regarding the EMS system.

Affective Objectives

1-1.6   Accept and uphold the responsibilities of a First Responder in accordance with the standards of an EMS professional.

1-1.7   Explain the rationale for maintaining a professional appearance when on duty or when responding to calls.

1-1.8   Describe why it is inappropriate to judge a patient based on a cultural, gender, age, or socioeconomic model, and to vary the standard of care rendered as a result of that judgement.

Psychomotor Objectives

No psychomotor objectives identified.

LESSON 1-2   THE WELL-BEING OF THE FIRST RESPONDER

Cognitive Objectives

At the completion of this lesson, the First Responder student will be able to:

1-2.1   List possible emotional reactions that the First Responder may experience when faced with trauma, illness, death, and dying.

1-2.2   Discuss the possible reactions that a family member may exhibit when confronted with death and dying.

1-2.3   State the steps in the First Responder's approach to the family confronted with death and dying.

1-2.4   State the possible reactions that the family of the First Responder may exhibit.

1-2.5   Recognize the signs and symptoms of critical-incident stress.

1-2.6   State possible steps that the First Responder may take to help reduce/alleviate stress.

1-2.7   Explain the need to determine scene safety.

1-2.8   Discuss the importance of body substance isolation (BSI).

1-2.9   Describe the steps the First Responder should take for personal protection from airborne and bloodborne pathogens.

1-2.10 List the personal protective equipment necessary for each of the following situations:
- Hazardous materials
- Rescue operations
- Violent scenes
- Crime scenes
- Electricity
- Water and ice
- Exposure to bloodborne pathogens
- Exposure to airborne pathogens

Affective Objectives

At the completion of this lesson, the First Responder student will be able to:

1-2.11 Explain the importance for serving as an advocate for the use of appropriate protective equipment.

1-2.12 Explain the importance of understanding the response to death and dying and communicating effectively with the patient's family.

1-2.13 Demonstrate a caring attitude toward any patient with illness or injury who requests emergency medical services.

1-2.14 Show compassion when caring for the physical and mental needs of patients.

1-2.15 Participate willingly in the care of all patients.

1-2.16 Communicate with empathy to patients being cared for, as well as to family members and friends of the patient.

Psychomotor Objectives

At the completion of this lesson, the First Responder student will be able to:

1-2.17 Given a scenario with potential infectious exposure, the First Responder will use appropriate personal protective equipment. At the completion of the scenario, the First Responder will properly remove and discard the protective garments.

1-2.18 Given the above scenario, the First Responder will complete disinfection/cleaning and all reporting documentation.

LESSON 1-3 LEGAL AND ETHICAL ISSUES

Cognitive Objectives

At the completion of this lesson, the First Responder student will be able to:

1-3.1 Define the First Responder scope of care.

1-3.2 Discuss the importance of Do Not Resuscitate [DNR] (advance directives) and local or state provisions regarding EMS application.

1-3.3 Define consent and discuss the methods of obtaining consent.

1-3.4 Differentiate between expressed and implied consent.

1-3.5 Explain the role of consent of minors in providing care.

1-3.6 Discuss the implications for the First Responder in patient refusal of transport.

1-3.7 Discuss the issues of abandonment, negligence, and battery and their implications to the First Responder.

1-3.8 State the conditions necessary for the First Responder to have a duty to act.

1-3.9 Explain the importance, necessity, and legality of patient confidentiality.

1-3.10 List the actions that a First Responder should take to assist in the preservation of a crime scene.

1-3.11 State the conditions that require a First Responder to notify local law enforcement officials.

1-3.12 Discuss issues concerning the fundamental components of documentation.

Affective Objectives

At the completion of this lesson, the First Responder student will be able to:

1-3.13 Explain the rationale for the needs, benefits and usage of advance directives.

1-3.14 Explain the rationale for the concept of varying degrees of DNR.

Psychomotor Objectives

No psychomotor objectives identified.

LESSON 1-4 THE HUMAN BODY
Cognitive Objectives
At the completion of this lesson, the First Responder student will be able to:

1-4.1   Describe the anatomy and function of the respiratory system.

1-4.2   Describe the anatomy and function of the circulatory system.

1-4.3   Describe the anatomy and function of the musculoskeletal system.

1-4.4   Describe the components and function of the nervous system.

Affective Objectives
No affective objectives identified.

Psychomotor Objectives
No psychomotor objectives identified.

LESSON 1-5 LIFTING AND MOVING PATIENTS
Cognitive Objectives
At the completion of this lesson, the First Responder student will be able to:

1-5.1   Define body mechanics.

1-5.2   Discuss the guidelines and safety precautions that need to be followed when lifting a patient.

1-5.3   Describe the indications for an emergency move.

1-5.4   Describe the indications for assisting in nonemergency moves.

1-5.5   Discuss the various devices associated with moving a patient in the out-of-hospital arena.

Affective Objectives
At the completion of this lesson, the First Responder student will be able to:

1-5.6   Explain the rationale for properly lifting and moving patients.

1-5.7   Explain the rationale for an emergency move.

Psychomotor Objectives
At the completion of this lesson, the First Responder student will be able to:

1-5.8   Demonstrate an emergency move.

1-5.9   Demonstrate a nonemergency move.

1-5.10 Demonstrate the use of equipment utilized to move patients in the out-of-hospital arena.

LESSON 1-6 EVALUATION: PREPARATORY
Cognitive Objectives
At the completion of this lesson, the First Responder student will be able to:

•   Demonstrate competence in the cognitive objectives of Lesson 1-1: Introduction to EMS Systems.

•   Demonstrate competence in the cognitive objectives of Lesson 1-2: The Well-Being of the First Responder.

•   Demonstrate competence in the cognitive objectives of Lesson 1-3: Legal and Ethical Issues.

•   Demonstrate competence in the cognitive objectives of Lesson 1-4: The Human Body.

•   Demonstrate competence in the cognitive objectives of Lesson 1-5: Lifting and Moving Patients.

Affective Objectives
At the completion of this lesson, the First Responder student will be able to:

•   Demonstrate competence in the affective objectives of Lesson 1-1: Introduction to EMS Systems.

•   Demonstrate competence in the affective objectives of Lesson 1-2: The Well-Being of the First Responder.

•   Demonstrate competence in the affective objectives of Lesson 1-3: Legal and Ethical Issues.

•   Demonstrate competence in the affective objectives of Lesson 1-4: The Human Body.

•   Demonstrate competence in the affective objectives of Lesson 1-5: Lifting and Moving Patients.

Psychomotor Objectives
At the completion of this lesson, the First Responder student will be able to:

•   Demonstrate competence in the psychomotor objectives of Lesson 1-1: Introduction to EMS Systems.

•   Demonstrate competence in the psychomotor objectives of Lesson 1-2: The Well-Being of the First Responder.

- Demonstrate competence in the psychomotor objectives of Lesson 1-3: Legal and Ethical Issues.
- Demonstrate competence in the psychomotor objectives of Lesson 1-4: The Human Body.
- Demonstrate competence in the psychomotor objectives of Lesson 1-5: Lifting and Moving Patients.

MODULE 2 AIRWAY

LESSON 2-1 AIRWAY
Cognitive Objectives
At the completion of this lesson, the First Responder student will be able to:

2-1.1   Name and label the major structures of the respiratory system on a diagram.

2-1.2   List the signs of inadequate breathing.

2-1.3   Describe the steps in the head-tilt, chin-lift.

2-1.4   Relate mechanism of injury to opening the airway.

2-1.5   Describe the steps in the jaw thrust.

2-1.6   State the importance of having a suction unit ready for immediate use when providing emergency medical care.

2-1.7   Describe the techniques of suctioning.

2-1.8   Describe how to ventilate a patient with a resuscitation mask or barrier device.

2-1.9   Describe how ventilating an infant or child is different from ventilating an adult.

2-1.10   List the steps in providing mouth-to-mouth and mouth-to-stoma ventilation.

2-1.11   Describe how to measure and insert an oropharyngeal (oral) airway.

2-1.12   Describe how to measure and insert an nasopharyngeal (nasal) airway.

2-1.13   Describe how to clear a foreign body airway obstruction in a responsive adult.

2-1.14   Describe how to clear a foreign body airway obstruction in a responsive child with complete obstruction or partial airway obstruction and poor air exchange.

2-1.15   Describe how to clear a foreign body airway obstruction in a responsive infant with complete obstruction or partial airway obstruction and poor air exchange.

2-1.16   Describe how to clear a foreign body airway obstruction in an unresponsive adult.

2-1.17   Describe how to clear a foreign body airway obstruction in an unresponsive child.

2-1.18   Describe how to clear a foreign body airway obstruction in an unresponsive infant.

Affective Objectives
At the completion of this lesson, the First Responder student will be able to:

2-1.19   Explain why basic life support ventilation and airway protective skills take priority over most other basic life support skills.

2-1.20   Demonstrate a caring attitude toward patients with airway problems who request emergency medical services.

2-1.21   Place the interests of the patient with airway problems as the foremost consideration when making any and all patient-care decisions.

2-1.22   Communicate with empathy to patients with airway problems, as well as to family members and friends of the patient.

Psychomotor Objectives
At the completion of this lesson, the First Responder student will be able to:

2-1.23   Demonstrate the steps in the head-tilt, chin-lift.

2-1.24   Demonstrate the steps in the jaw thrust.

2-1.25   Demonstrate the techniques of suctioning.

2-1.26   Demonstrate the steps in mouth-to-mouth ventilation with body substance isolation (barrier shields).

2-1.27   Demonstrate how to use a resuscitation mask to ventilate a patient.

2-1.28   Demonstrate how to ventilate a patient with a stoma.

2-1.29   Demonstrate how to measure and insert an oropharyngeal (oral) airway.

2-1.30   Demonstrate how to measure and insert a nasopharyngeal (nasal) airway.

2-1.31   Demonstrate how to ventilate infant and child patients.

2-1.32   Demonstrate how to clear a foreign body airway obstruction in a responsive adult.

2-1.33   Demonstrate how to clear a foreign body airway obstruction in a responsive child.

2-1.34   Demonstrate how to clear a foreign body airway obstruction in a responsive infant.

2-1.35   Demonstrate how to clear a foreign body airway obstruction in an unresponsive adult.

2-1.36   Demonstrate how to clear a foreign body airway obstruction in an unresponsive child.

2-1.37   Demonstrate how to clear a foreign body airway obstruction in an unresponsive infant.

LESSON 2-2   PRACTICAL LAB: AIRWAY
Cognitive Objectives

At the completion of this lesson, the First Responder student will be able to:

- Demonstrate the cognitive objectives of Lesson 2-1: Airway.

Affective Objectives

At the completion of this lesson, the First Responder student will be able to:

- Demonstrate the affective objectives of Lesson 2-1: Airway.

Psychomotor Objectives

At the completion of this lesson, the First Responder student will be able to:

- Demonstrate the steps in the head-tilt, chin-lift.
- Demonstrate the steps in the jaw thrust.
- Demonstrate the techniques of suctioning.
- Demonstrate the steps in mouth-to-mouth ventilation with body substance isolation (barrier shields).
- Demonstrate how to use a resuscitation mask to ventilate a patient.
- Demonstrate how to ventilate a patient with a stoma.
- Demonstrate how to measure and insert an oropharyngeal (oral) airway.
- Demonstrate how to measure and insert a nasopharyngeal (nasal) airway.
- Demonstrate how to ventilate infant and child patients.
- Demonstrate how to clear a foreign body airway obstruction in a responsive adult.

- Demonstrate how to clear a foreign body airway obstruction in a responsive child.
- Demonstrate how to clear a foreign body airway obstruction in a responsive infant.
- Demonstrate how to clear a foreign body airway obstruction in an unresponsive adult.
- Demonstrate how to clear a foreign body airway obstruction in an unresponsive child.
- Demonstrate how to clear a foreign body airway obstruction in an unresponsive infant.

LESSON 2-3   EVALUATION: AIRWAY
Cognitive Objectives

At the completion of this lesson, the First Responder student will be able to:

- Demonstrate competence in the cognitive objectives of Lesson 2-1: Airway.

Affective Objectives

At the completion of this lesson, the First Responder student will be able to:

- Demonstrate competence in the affective objectives of Lesson 2-1: Airway.

Psychomotor Objectives

At the completion of this lesson, the First Responder student will be able to:

- Demonstrate competence in the psychomotor objectives of Lesson 2-1: Airway.

MODULE 3   PATIENT ASSESSMENT

LESSON 3-1   PATIENT ASSESSMENT
Cognitive Objectives

At the completion of this lesson, the First Responder student will be able to:

3-1.1   Discuss the components of scene size-up.

3-1.2   Describe common hazards found at the scene of a trauma and a medical patient.

3-1.3   Determine if the scene is safe to enter.

3-1.4   Discuss common mechanisms of injury/nature of illness.

3-1.5   Discuss the reason for identifying the total number of patients at the scene.

3-1.6   Explain the reason for identifying the need for additional help or assistance.

3-1.7   Summarize the reasons for forming a general impression of the patient.

3-1.8   Discuss methods of assessing mental status.

3-1.9 Differentiate between assessing mental status in the adult, child, and infant patient.

3-1.10 Describe methods used for assessing if a patient is breathing.

3-1.11 Differentiate between a patient with adequate and inadequate breathing.

3-1.12 Describe the methods used to assess circulation.

3-1.13 Differentiate among obtaining a pulse in an adult, child, and infant patient.

3-1.14 Discuss the need for assessing the patient for external bleeding.

3-1.15 Explain the reason for prioritizing a patient for care and transport.

3-1.16 Discuss the components of the physical exam.

3-1.17 State the areas of the body that are evaluated during the physical exam.

3-1.18 Explain what additional questioning may be asked during the physical exam.

3-1.19 Explain the components of the SAMPLE history.

3-1.20 Discuss the components of the ongoing assessment.

3-1.21 Describe the information included in the First Responder hand-off report.

Affective Objectives

At the completion of this lesson, the First Responder student will be able to:

3-1.22 Explain the rationale for crew members to evaluate scene safety prior to entering.

3-1.23 Serve as a model for others by explaining how patient situations affect your evaluation of the mechanism of injury or illness.

3-1.24 Explain the importance of forming a general impression of the patient.

3-1.25 Explain the value of an initial assessment.

3-1.26 Explain the value of questioning the patient and family.

3-1.27 Explain the value of the physical exam.

3-1.28 Explain the value of an ongoing assessment.

3-1.29 Explain the rationale for the feelings that these patients might be experiencing.

3-1.30 Demonstrate a caring attitude when performing patient assessments.

3-1.31 Place the interests of the patient as the foremost consideration when making any and all patient-care decisions during patient assessment.

3-1.32 Communicate with empathy during patient assessment to patients as well as to family members and friends of the patient.

Psychomotor Objectives

At the completion of this lesson, the First Responder student will be able to:

3-1.33 Demonstrate the ability to differentiate various scenarios and identify potential hazards.

3-1.34 Demonstrate the techniques for assessing mental status.

3-1.35 Demonstrate the techniques for assessing the airway.

3-1.36 Demonstrate the techniques for assessing if the patient is breathing.

3-1.37 Demonstrate the techniques for assessing if the patient has a pulse.

3-1.38 Demonstrate the techniques for assessing the patient for external bleeding.

3-1.39 Demonstrate the techniques for assessing the patient's skin color, temperature, condition, and capillary refill (infants and children only).

3-1.40 Demonstrate questioning a patient to obtain a SAMPLE history.

3-1.41 Demonstrate the skills involved in performing the physical exam.

3-1.42 Demonstrate the ongoing assessment.

LESSON 3-2 PRACTICAL LAB: PATIENT ASSESSMENT
Cognitive Objectives

At the completion of this lesson, the First Responder student will be able to:

• Demonstrate the cognitive objectives of Lesson 3-1: Patient Assessment.

Affective Objectives

At the completion of this lesson, the First Responder student will be able to:

• Demonstrate the affective objectives of Lesson 3-1: Patient Assessment.

Psychomotor Objectives

At the completion of this lesson, the First Responder student will be able to:

- Demonstrate the ability to differentiate various scenarios and identify potential hazards.
- Demonstrate the techniques for assessing mental status.
- Demonstrate the techniques for assessing the airway.
- Demonstrate the techniques for assessing if the patient is breathing.
- Demonstrate the techniques for assessing if the patient has a pulse.
- Demonstrate the techniques for assessing the patient for external bleeding.
- Demonstrate the techniques for assessing the patient's skin color, temperature, condition, and capillary refill (infants and children only).
- Demonstrate questioning a patient to obtain a SAMPLE history.
- Demonstrate the skills involved in performing the physical exam.
- Demonstrate the ongoing assessment.

LESSON 3-3   EVALUATION: PATIENT ASSESSMENT

Cognitive Objectives

At the completion of this lesson, the First Responder student will be able to:

- Demonstrate competence in the cognitive objectives of Lesson 3-1: Patient Assessment.

Affective Objectives

At the completion of this lesson, the First Responder student will be able to:

- Demonstrate competence in the affective objectives of Lesson 3-1: Patient Assessment.

Psychomotor Objectives

At the completion of this lesson, the First Responder student will be able to:

- Demonstrate competence in the psychomotor objectives of Lesson 3-1: Patient Assessment.

MODULE 4   CIRCULATION

LESSON 4-1   CIRCULATION

Cognitive Objectives

At the completion of this lesson, the First Responder student will be able to:

4-1.1   List the reasons for the heart to stop beating.

4-1.2   Define the components of cardiopulmonary resuscitation.

4-1.3   Describe each link in the chain of survival and how it relates to the EMS system.

4-1.4   List the steps of one-rescuer adult CPR.

4-1.5   Describe the technique of external chest compressions on an adult patient.

4-1.6   Describe the technique of external chest compressions on an infant.

4-1.7   Describe the technique of external chest compressions on a child.

4-1.8   Explain when the First Responder is able to stop CPR.

4-1.9   List the steps of two-rescuer adult CPR.

4-1.10   List the steps of infant CPR.

4-1.11   List the steps of child CPR.

Affective Objectives

At the completion of this lesson, the First Responder student will be able to:

4-1.12   Respond to the feelings that the family of a patient may be having during a cardiac event.

4-1.13   Demonstrate a caring attitude toward patients with cardiac events who request emergency medical services.

4-1.14   Place the interests of the patient with a cardiac event as the foremost consideration when making any and all patient-care decisions.

4-1.15   Communicate with empathy with family members and friends of the patient with a cardiac event.

Psychomotor Objectives

At the completion of this lesson, the First Responder student will be able to:

4-1.16   Demonstrate the proper technique of chest compressions on an adult.

4-1.17   Demonstrate the proper technique of chest compressions on a child.

4-1.18   Demonstrate the proper technique of chest compressions on an infant.

4-1.19   Demonstrate the steps of adult one-rescuer CPR.

4-1.20   Demonstrate the steps of adult two-rescuer CPR.

4-1.21   Demonstrate child CPR.

4-1.22   Demonstrate infant CPR.

LESSON 4-2 PRACTICAL LAB: CIRCULATION

Cognitive Objectives

At the completion of this lesson, the First Responder student will be able to:

- Demonstrate the cognitive objectives of Lesson 4-1: Circulation.

Affective Objectives

At the completion of this lesson, the First Responder student will be able to:

- Demonstrate the affective objectives of Lesson 4-1: Circulation.

Psychomotor Objectives

At the completion of this lesson, the First Responder student will be able to:

- Demonstrate the proper technique of chest compressions on an adult.
- Demonstrate the proper technique of chest compressions on a child.
- Demonstrate the proper technique of chest compressions on an infant.
- Demonstrate the steps of adult one-rescuer CPR.
- Demonstrate the steps of adult two-rescuer CPR.
- Demonstrate child CPR.
- Demonstrate infant CPR.

LESSON 4-3 EVALUATION: CIRCULATION

Cognitive Objectives

At the completion of this lesson, the First Responder student will be able to:

- Demonstrate competence in the cognitive objectives of Lesson 4-1: Circulation.
- Demonstrate competence in the cognitive objectives of Lesson 4-2: Circulation.

Affective Objectives

At the completion of this lesson, the First Responder student will be able to:

- Demonstrate competence in the affective objectives of Lesson 4-1: Circulation.
- Demonstrate competence in the affective objectives of Lesson 4-2: Circulation.

Psychomotor Objectives

At the completion of this lesson, the First Responder student will be able to:

- Demonstrate competence in the psychomotor objectives of Lesson 4-1: Circulation.

- Demonstrate competence in the psychomotor objectives of Lesson 4-2: Circulation.

MODULE 5 ILLNESS AND INJURY

LESSON 5-1 MEDICAL EMERGENCIES

Cognitive Objectives

At the completion of this lesson, the First Responder student will be able to:

5-1.1 Identify the patient who presents with a general medical complaint.

5-1.2 Explain the steps in providing emergency medical care to a patient with a general medical complaint.

5-1.3 Identify the patient who presents with a specific medical complaint of altered mental status.

5-1.4 Explain the steps in providing emergency medical care to a patient with an altered mental status.

5-1.5 Identify the patient who presents with a specific medical complaint of seizures.

5-1.6 Explain the steps in providing emergency medical care to a patient with seizures.

5-1.7 Identify the patient who presents with a specific medical complaint of exposure to cold.

5-1.8 Explain the steps in providing emergency medical care to a patient with an exposure to cold.

5-1.9 Identify the patient who presents with a specific medical complaint of exposure to heat.

5-1.10 Explain the steps in providing emergency medical care to a patient with an exposure to heat.

5-1.11 Identify the patient who presents with a specific medical complaint of behavioral change.

5-1.12 Explain the steps in providing emergency medical care to a patient with a behavioral change.

5-1.13 Identify the patient who presents with a specific complaint of a psychological crisis.

5-1.14 Explain the steps in providing emergency medical care to a patient with a psychological crisis.

Affective Objectives

At the completion of this lesson, the First Responder student will be able to:

5-1.15 Attend to the feelings of the patient and/or family when dealing with the patient with a general medical complaint.

5-1.16 Attend to the feelings of the patient and/or family when dealing with the patient with a specific medical complaint.

5-1.17 Explain the rationale for modifying your behavior toward the patient with a behavioral emergency.

5-1.18 Demonstrate a caring attitude toward patients with a general medical complaint who request emergency medical services.

5-1.19 Place the interests of the patient with a general medical complaint as the foremost consideration when making any and all patient-care decisions.

5-1.20 Communicate with empathy to patients with a general medical complaint, as well as to family members and friends of the patient.

5-1.21 Demonstrate a caring attitude toward patients with a specific medical complaint who request emergency medical services.

5-1.22 Place the interests of the patient with a specific medical complaint as the foremost consideration when making any and all patient-care decisions.

5-1.23 Communicate with empathy to patients with a specific medical complaint, as well as to family members and friends of the patient.

5-1.24 Demonstrate a caring attitude toward patients with a behavioral problem who request emergency medical services.

5-1.25 Place the interests of the patient with a behavioral problem as the foremost consideration when making any and all patient-care decisions.

5-1.26 Communicate with empathy to patients with a behavioral problem, as well as to family members and friends of the patient.

Psychomotor Objectives

At the completion of this lesson, the First Responder student will be able to:

5-1.27 Demonstrate the steps in providing emergency medical care to a patient with a general medical complaint.

5-1.28 Demonstrate the steps in providing emergency medical care to a patient with an altered mental status.

5-1.29 Demonstrate the steps in providing emergency medical care to a patient with seizures.

5-1.30 Demonstrate the steps in providing emergency medical care to a patient with an exposure to cold.

5-1.31 Demonstrate the steps in providing emergency medical care to a patient with an exposure to heat.

5-1.32 Demonstrate the steps in providing emergency medical care to a patient with a behavioral change.

5-1.33 Demonstrate the steps in providing emergency medical care to a patient with a psychological crisis.

LESSON 5-2   BLEEDING AND SOFT-TISSUE INJURIES

Cognitive Objectives

At the completion of this lesson, the First Responder student will be able to:

5-2.1 Differentiate between arterial, venous, and capillary bleeding.

5-2.2 State the emergency medical care for external bleeding.

5-2.3 Establish the relationship between body substance isolation and bleeding.

5-2.4 List the signs of internal bleeding.

5-2.5 List the steps in the emergency medical care of the patient with signs and symptoms of internal bleeding.

5-2.6 Establish the relationship between body substance isolation (BSI) and soft-tissue injuries.

5-2.7 State the types of open soft-tissue injuries.

5-2.8 Describe the emergency medical care of the patient with a soft-tissue injury.

5-2.9 Discuss the emergency medical care considerations for a patient with a penetrating chest injury.

5-2.10 State the emergency medical care considerations for a patient with an open wound to the abdomen.

5-2.11 Describe the emergency medical care for an impaled object.

5-2.12 State the emergency medical care for an amputation.

5-2.13 Describe the emergency medical care for burns.

5-2.14 List the functions of dressing and bandaging.

Affective Objectives

At the completion of this lesson, the First Responder student will be able to:

5-2.15 Explain the rationale for body substance isolation when dealing with bleeding and soft-tissue injuries.

5-2.16 Attend to the feelings of the patient with a soft-tissue injury or bleeding.

5-2.17 Demonstrate a caring attitude toward patients with a soft-tissue injury or bleeding who request emergency medical services.

5-2.18 Place the interests of the patient with a soft-tissue injury or bleeding as the foremost consideration when making any and all patient-care decisions.

5-2.19 Communicate with empathy to patients with a soft-tissue injury or bleeding, as well as with family members and friends of the patient.

Psychomotor Objectives

At the completion of this lesson, the First Responder student will be able to:

5-2.20 Demonstrate direct pressure as a method of emergency medical care for external bleeding.

5-2.21 Demonstrate the use of diffuse pressure as a method of emergency medical care for external bleeding.

5-2.22 Demonstrate the use of pressure points as a method of emergency medical care for external bleeding.

5-2.23 Demonstrate the care of the patient exhibiting signs and symptoms of internal bleeding.

5-2.24 Demonstrate the steps in the emergency medical care of open soft-tissue injuries.

5-2.25 Demonstrate the steps in the emergency medical care of a patient with an open chest wound.

5-2.26 Demonstrate the steps in the emergency medical care of a patient with open abdominal wounds.

5-2.27 Demonstrate the steps in the emergency medical care of a patient with an impaled object.

5-2.28 Demonstrate the steps in the emergency medical care of a patient with an amputation.

5-2.29 Demonstrate the steps in the emergency medical care of an amputated part.

LESSON 5-3 INJURIES TO MUSCLES AND BONES

Cognitive Objectives

At the completion of this lesson, the First Responder student will be able to:

5-3.1 Describe the function of the musculoskeletal system.

5-3.2 Differentiate between an open and a closed painful, swollen, deformed extremity.

5-3.3 List the emergency medical care for a patient with a painful, swollen, deformed extremity.

5-3.4 Relate mechanism of injury to potential injuries of the head and spine.

5-3.5 State the signs and symptoms of a potential spine injury.

5-3.6 Describe the method of determining if a responsive patient may have a spine injury.

5-3.7 List the signs and symptoms of injury to the head.

5-3.8 Describe the emergency medical care for injuries to the head.

Affective Objectives

At the completion of this lesson, the First Responder student will be able to:

5-3.9 Explain the rationale for the feeling patients who have need for immobilization of the painful, swollen, deformed extremity.

5-3.10 Demonstrate a caring attitude toward patients with a musculoskeletal injury who request emergency medical services.

5-3.11 Place the interests of the patient with a musculoskeletal injury as the foremost consideration when making any and all patient-care decisions.

5-3.12 Communicate with empathy to patients with a musculoskeletal injury, as well as to family members and friends of the patient.

Psychomotor Objectives

At the completion of this lesson, the First Responder student will be able to:

5-3.13 Demonstrate the emergency medical care of a patient with a painful, swollen, deformed extremity.

5-3.14 Demonstrate opening the airway in a patient with a suspected spinal cord injury.

5-3.15 Demonstrate evaluating a responsive patient with a suspected spinal cord injury.

5-3.16 Demonstrate stabilizing of the cervical spine.

Lesson 5-4 Practical Lab: Illness and Injury

Cognitive Objectives

At the completion of this lesson, the First Responder student will be able to:

- Demonstrate the cognitive objectives of Lesson 5-1: Medical Emergencies.
- Demonstrate the cognitive objectives of Lesson 5-2: Bleeding and Soft-Tissue Injuries.
- Demonstrate the cognitive objectives of Lesson 5-3: Injuries to Muscles and Bones.

Affective Objectives

At the completion of this lesson, the First Responder student will be able to:

- Demonstrate the affective objectives of Lesson 5-1: Medical Emergencies.

- Demonstrate the affective objectives of Lesson 5-2: Bleeding and Soft-Tissue Injuries.
- Demonstrate the affective objectives of Lesson 5-3: Injuries to Muscles and Bones.

Psychomotor Objectives

At the completion of this lesson, the First Responder student will be able to:

- Demonstrate the steps in providing emergency medical care to a patient with a general medical complaint.
- Demonstrate the steps in providing emergency medical care to a patient with an altered mental status.
- Demonstrate the steps in providing emergency medical care to a patient with seizures.
- Demonstrate the steps in providing emergency medical care to a patient with an exposure to cold.
- Demonstrate the steps in providing emergency medical care to a patient with an exposure to heat.
- Demonstrate the steps in providing emergency medical care to a patient with a behavioral change.
- Demonstrate the steps in providing emergency medical care to a patient with a psychological crisis.
- Demonstrate direct pressure as a method of emergency medical care for external bleeding.
- Demonstrate the use of diffuse pressure as a method of emergency medical care for external bleeding.
- Demonstrate the use of pressure points as a method of emergency medical care for external bleeding.
- Demonstrate the care of the patient exhibiting signs and symptoms of internal bleeding.
- Demonstrate the steps in the emergency medical care of open soft-tissue injuries.
- Demonstrate the steps in the emergency medical care of a patient with an open chest wound.
- Demonstrate the steps in the emergency medical care of a patient with open abdominal wounds.

- Demonstrate the steps in the emergency medical care of a patient with an impaled object.
- Demonstrate the steps in the emergency medical care of a patient with an amputation.
- Demonstrate the steps in the emergency medical care of an amputated part.
- Demonstrate the emergency medical care of a patient with a painful, swollen, deformed extremity.
- Demonstrate opening the airway in a patient with a suspected spinal cord injury.
- Demonstrate evaluating a responsive patient with a suspected spinal cord injury.
- Demonstrate stabilizing of the cervical spine.

LESSON 5-5 EVALUATION: ILLNESS AND INJURY

Cognitive Objectives

At the completion of this lesson, the First Responder student will be able to:

- Demonstrate competence in the cognitive objectives of Lesson 5-1: Medical Emergencies.
- Demonstrate competence in the cognitive objectives of Lesson 5-2: Bleeding and Soft-Tissue Injuries.
- Demonstrate competence in the cognitive objectives of Lesson 5-3: Injuries to Muscles and Bones.

Affective Objectives

At the completion of this lesson, the First Responder student will be able to:

- Demonstrate competence in the affective objectives of Lesson 5-1: Medical Emergencies.
- Demonstrate competence in the affective objectives of Lesson 5-2: Bleeding and Soft-Tissue Injuries.
- Demonstrate competence in the affective objectives of Lesson 5-3: Injuries to Muscles and Bones.

Psychomotor Objectives

At the completion of this lesson, the First Responder student will be able to:

- Demonstrate competence in the psychomotor objectives of Lesson 5-1: Medical Emergencies.

- Demonstrate competence in the psychomotor objectives of Lesson 5-2: Bleeding and Soft-Tissue Injuries.
- Demonstrate competence in the psychomotor objectives of Lesson 5-3: Injuries to Muscles and Bones.

MODULE 6 CHILDBIRTH AND CHILDREN

LESSON 6-1 CHILDBIRTH

Cognitive Objectives

At the completion of this lesson, the First Responder student will be able to:

6-1.1 Identify the following structures: birth canal, placenta, umbilical cord, amniotic sac.

6-1.2 Define the following terms: crowning, bloody show, labor, abortion.

6-1.3 State indications of an imminent delivery.

6-1.4 State the steps in the predelivery preparation of the mother.

6-1.5 Establish the relationship between body substance isolation and childbirth.

6-1.6 State the steps to assist in the delivery.

6-1.7 Describe care of the baby as the head appears.

6-1.8 Discuss the steps in delivery of the placenta.

6-1.9 List the steps in the emergency medical care of the mother post-delivery.

6-1.10 Discuss the steps in caring for a newborn.

Affective Objectives

At the completion of this lesson, the First Responder student will be able to:

6-1.11 Explain the rationale for attending to the feelings of a patient in need of emergency medical care during childbirth.

6-1.12 Demonstrate a caring attitude toward patients during childbirth who request emergency medical services.

6-1.13 Place the interests of the patient during childbirth as the foremost consideration when making any and all patient-care decisions.

6-1.14 Communicate with empathy to patients during childbirth, as well as to family members and friends of the patient.

Psychomotor Objectives

At the completion of this lesson, the First Responder student will be able to:

6-1.15 Demonstrate the steps to assist in the normal cephalic delivery.

6-1.16 Demonstrate necessary care procedures of the fetus as the head appears.

6-1.17 Attend to the steps in the delivery of the placenta.

6-1.18 Demonstrate the post-delivery care of the mother.

6-1.19 Demonstrate the care of the newborn.

LESSON 6-2 INFANTS AND CHILDREN

Cognitive Objectives

At the completion of this lesson, the First Responder student will be able to:

6-2.1 Describe differences in anatomy and physiology of the infant, child, and adult patient.

6-2.2 Describe assessment of the infant or child.

6-2.3 Indicate various causes of respiratory emergencies in infants and children.

6-2.4 Summarize emergency medical care strategies for respiratory distress and respiratory failure/arrest in infants and children.

6-2.5 List common causes of seizures in the infant and child patient.

6-2.6 Describe management of seizures in the infant and child patient.

6-2.7 Discuss emergency medical care of the infant and child trauma patient.

6-2.8 Summarize the signs and symptoms of possible child abuse and neglect.

6-2.9 Describe the medical-legal responsibilities in suspected child abuse.

6-2.10 Recognize need for First Responder debriefing following a difficult infant or child transport.

Affective Objectives

At the completion of this lesson, the First Responder student will be able to:

6-2.11 Attend to the feelings of the family when dealing with an ill or injured infant or child.

6-2.12 Understand the provider's own emotional response to caring for infants or children.

6-2.13 Demonstrate a caring attitude toward infants and children with illness or injury who require emergency medical services.

6-2.14 Place the interests of the infant or child with an illness or injury as the foremost consideration when making any and all patient-care decisions.

6-2.15 Communicate with empathy to infants and children with an illness or injury, as well as to family members and friends of the patient.

Psychomotor Objectives

At the completion of this lesson, the First Responder student will be able to:

6-2.16 Demonstrate assessment of the infant and child.

LESSON 6-3 PRACTICAL LAB: CHILDBIRTH AND CHILDREN

Cognitive Objectives

At the completion of this lesson, the First Responder student will be able to:

• Demonstrate the cognitive objectives of Lesson 6-1: Childbirth.

• Demonstrate the cognitive objectives of Lesson 6-2: Infants and Children.

Affective Objectives

At the completion of this lesson, the First Responder student will be able to:

• Demonstrate the affective objectives of Lesson 6-1: Childbirth.

• Demonstrate the affective objectives of Lesson 6-2: Infants and Children.

Psychomotor Objectives

At the completion of this lesson, the First Responder student will be able to:

• Demonstrate the steps to assist in the normal cephalic delivery.

• Demonstrate necessary care procedures of the fetus as the head appears.

• Attend to the steps in the delivery of the placenta.

• Demonstrate the post-delivery care of the mother.

• Demonstrate the care of the newborn.

• Demonstrate assessment of the infant and child.

LESSON 6-4   EVALUATION: CHILDBIRTH AND CHILDREN

Cognitive Objectives

At the completion of this lesson, the First Responder student will be able to:

- Demonstrate competence in the cognitive objectives of Lesson 6-1: Childbirth.
- Demonstrate competence in the cognitive objectives of Lesson 6-2: Infants and Children.

Affective Objectives

At the completion of this lesson, the First Responder student will be able to:

- Demonstrate competence in the affective objectives of Lesson 6-1: Childbirth.
- Demonstrate competence in the affective objectives of Lesson 6-2: Infants and Children.

Psychomotor Objectives

At the completion of this lesson, the First Responder student will be able to:

- Demonstrate competence in the psychomotor objectives of Lesson 6-1: Childbirth.
- Demonstrate competence in the psychomotor objectives of Lesson 6-2: Infants and Children.

MODULE 7   EMS OPERATIONS

LESSON 7-1   EMS OPERATIONS

Cognitive Objectives

At the completion of this lesson, the First Responder student will be able to:

7-1.1   Discuss the medical and nonmedical equipment needed to respond to a call.

7-1.2   List the phases of an out-of-hospital call.

7-1.3   Discuss the role of the First Responder in extrication.

7-1.4   List various methods of gaining access to the patient.

7-1.5   Distinguish between simple and complex access.

7-1.6   Describe what the First Responder should do if there is reason to believe that there is a hazard at the scene.

7-1.7   State the role the First Responder should perform until appropriately trained personnel arrive at the scene of a hazardous materials situation.

7-1.8   Describe the criteria for a multiple-casualty situation.

7-1.9   Discuss the role of the First Responder in the multiple-casualty situation.

7-1.10   Summarize the components of basic triage.

Affective Objectives

At the completion of this lesson, the First Responder student will be able to:

7-1.11   Explain the rationale for having the unit prepared to respond.

Psychomotor Objectives

At the completion of this lesson, the First Responder student will be able to:

7-1.12   Given a scenario of a mass-casualty incident, perform triage.

LESSON 7-2   EVALUATION: EMS OPERATIONS

Cognitive Objectives

At the completion of this lesson, the First Responder student will be able to:

- Demonstrate competence in the cognitive objectives of Lesson 7-1: EMS Operations.

Affective Objectives

At the completion of this lesson, the First Responder student will be able to:

- Demonstrate competence in the affective objectives of Lesson 7-1: EMS Operations.

Psychomotor Objectives

At the completion of this lesson, the First Responder student will be able to:

- Demonstrate competence in the psychomotor objectives of Lesson 7-1: EMS Operations.

Index